BABY SLEEP TRAINING

TABLE OF CONTENTS

INTRODUCTION

The first month of life is exhausting for parents. Your baby can't tell the difference between day and night and needs to be fed every two to four hours. But once you're through that initial rough patch, it is possible to teach her to sleep through the night. Sleep in infancy, and in particular sleep training, is an area that is so riddled with confusion and controversy.

People who don't have sleep issues may think the idea of 'teaching' a child to fall asleep is ridiculous. What many people do not know is that falling asleep unassisted, like many other behaviours, is a skill that is learned. And just like anything in parenting, if you want to teach your child a new skill, it is going to require time, patience and a ton of consistency.

Sleep training, or helping your baby learn good sleep habits and how to sleep more independently, can be the source of many questions. One of the most pressing questions is what sleep training method is right for your baby. This book will cover the 5 most common sleep training methods though there are many variations within each method that you can customize for your baby.

One common misconception about sleep training babies (also called sleep coaching) is that there's only one way to do it. But this could not be further from the truth! In reality, there are a number of ways many parents can work to help their babies develop healthy sleep habits and stop waking up in the middle of the night or taking short naps. Some methods involve crying, but others involve little to no tears and are very gentle.

So what methods should you try with your baby? To help you answer that question, we've created a baby sleep training 'cheat sheet', complete with a list of the most common sleep training methods as well as explanations of how they work.

Toddlers who wake up during the middle of the night often get used to having a parent or caretaker help soothe them back to sleep. However, this can eventually develop into a pattern of being unable to fall back asleep on their own, which ends up robbing both the child and the adult of much needed rest. Teaching a toddler to fall back asleep on their own at night will result in more sleep for everyone.

CHAPTER ONE

Better Sleep for your Baby

The ideas in this pack are for any parent who is thinking about ways to help their baby, their child or themself to get more sleep, particularly at night. During the first months of life, it is normal for babies to wake frequently at night. Night feeding is important for babies' growth and for establishing breastfeeding. It is important to babies' development that their parents respond to their needs for company, comfort and food.

As children get older, they begin to separate night from day until they reach an age when they can sleep all night. Sleep training is not recommended in the first few months, but many parents find it helpful to encourage independent settling and to introduce bedtime routines for their babies, to set the scene for good sleep later on. Some of the ideas in this pack will be useful to most parents. Some might only be useful for a parent who wants to make a big change to their child's sleep pattern. Some techniques are suitable for babies, some are suitable for toddlers and older children.

All families are different. What suits one family will not suit another. Some parents are happy for their babies to stay up late and to wake frequently. Other parents find their child's night waking difficult and want to make changes. There is no right approach when it comes to sleep. Some sleep training techniques are gentle and are unlikely to upset children or their parents. These techniques can take hours every evening to implement and may take several weeks to be effective. Other sleep training techniques are likely to involve some crying which may get worse before it gets better. These can be distressing but are usually effective within a week and can be helpful when parents want a major change.

Some babies sleep in cots at night, others sleep in their parents' beds. Babies may have daytime naps in slings, bouncy chairs, prams, Moses baskets, cots. Sleep training techniques can be adapted to the different places your baby sleeps. Different techniques can work at different times in your child's life. What worked when they were a baby may not work when they are four years old. If what you have tried has not worked, your health visitor can carry out an assessment of your sleep situation and help you try a different approach.

Does your baby need to be rocked to sleep by you or wake up in the middle of the night demanding a breast, bottle or cuddle before drifting back to sleep? If your little one is at least 4 months old, it may be time to start sleep training.

By that age, babies can and should be able to fall asleep or fall back to sleep on their own by self-soothing.

If you're dreading sleep training (also called sleep teaching), know that it's often accomplished faster than many parents imagine, and it doesn't necessarily even have to involve lots of tears. Here's how and when to start sleep training your baby to help everyone get a good night's sleep.

What is Sleep Training?

Baby sleep coaching is a fairly new concept. A sleep coach is a professional who can aid you in teaching your baby the skills necessary to put themselves to sleep. A baby that is able to self soothe allows both the parents as well as other members of your household to have a more restful night's sleep. When you utilize the support of a baby sleep coach, you are taking a huge step towards restoring a more peaceful environment for you and your family.

If you have a new baby then you are aware of what a toll it can take on your own sleep patterns to have your baby waking many times throughout the night. As a loving new parent, you are often focused on providing your newborn with the feeling of love and security - but you have to take care of your own needs as well. You are not able to properly care for either yourself or your baby if you are not well rested.

All new parents suffer from some level of sleep deprivation at first, but if after four months you are still having trouble getting your baby to sleep you could definitely benefit from the aid of a baby sleep coach. They are trained to help with babies' sleep problems and can assist you and your family to get a good night's rest.

A baby sleep coach can be a great support in helping you teach your baby to develop healthy sleep habits. Unlike sitting up or rolling over, good sleep habits are not innate. Being able to put themselves to sleep is a skill most babies need assistance to learn. A baby sleep coach can be the greatest resource available to provide support and information so can help your baby get the sleep he or she needs for healthy development.

Once you've accepted that the expertise of a baby sleep coach could help restore some harmony to your family environment, you can decide if a phone or in home consultation will work best for you. During the initial consultation, the sleep coach will review your unique family situation. After inquiring about your feelings on various methods and assessing your baby's current sleep patterns, they will create a custom sleep plan and answer any questions you have about how to begin implementation.

If you have been struggling night after night with getting your baby to sleep or back to sleep, please know there is hope! Many parents feel a great sense of relief even after the first consultation. They soon realize they are not alone, and they can receive help with their baby's sleep problems, while having an experienced coach with them each step of the way.

What Sleep Training isn't

First, sleep training and night weaning do not necessarily go hand-in-hand. You can still feed your baby once or even twice during the night, depending on age and stage. Talk to your pediatrician about when it's appropriate to fully drop your baby's nighttime feeds.

That's one of many ways that sleep training is not as harsh as it sounds. It doesn't necessarily involve shutting the nursery door and letting baby cry all night. In fact, you can adjust the amount of crying you let your baby do to your comfort level before you offer a soothing song or a comforting rub on the back.

While some parents worry that some methods might harm a baby's health or create attachment-related issues down the line, research shows that sleep training doesn't increase the risk of behavioral or emotional problems later in childhood.

Many experts say that sleep training is not only safe, it's healthy and important for babies' development.

When should I Consider Sleep Training?

I would wait until a child is at least 6 months of age, although some people have recommended trying it as early as two month of age (note that I don't endorse this). I actually think that it is a bad idea to start before four months of age, preferably once he is no longer feeding during the night. However, if your child is still feeding multiple times during the night and is over six months of age, that could be part of the problem. If your child has issues such as autism or developmental delay, these techniques will still work but must be applied more slowly.

When should I not start Sleep Training?

If you are worried that your child may have a medical problem which is disrupting sleep, please talk to your pediatrician.

If you want to pursue co-sleeping as a lifestyle, you may find it more difficult to adopt these recommendations, although they can be put into play if you are room or even bedsharing– it is just harder. I believe that cosleeping is associated with worse sleep long term for parent and child. If you are cosleeping and want to stop, here is my guide on how to stop the cosleeping habit.

If you have a major life event coming up– a move, a visit from the in-laws, a big project do at work.

If you have major stresses in your that would make embarking on about a week of disruption.

Baby Sleeping - What Mothers Need To Know

During the early weeks, the baby's sleep will be affecting you. In fact, there are a lot of new parents often find themselves exhausted, frustrated, and wondering if their baby will ever sleep through the night. According to research, 20 percent of nine-month-old babies have difficulty in falling asleep and 42 percent awake at night. Sleep is not a habit that you can force your baby into. It must normally overtake your baby. At night, your role as a parent is to set the conditions that make sleep possible and to show signals that advise to baby that sleep is expected.

If your baby is frequently waking in the night it can affect your own sleep patterns and may cause you to be exhausted with your tasks the next day. Mothers with babies that have sleeping problems are prone to depression if they experience frequent sleep disturbances. It can also affect the relationship between you and your husband. Here is some tips to get your baby go to sleep.

Sleeping Tips For Mums

1. Give your baby a chance to fall asleep on his own from about six to eight weeks. Put him to bed when he's sleepy, but still awake. According to research, rocking or breastfeeding infants to sleep is not advisable because babies may come to depend on it.

2. You can make daytime feed fun and lively and night time feeds comfortable and quiet. This strategy can help you set her body clock so the baby can learn the difference between day and night.

3. You can play music. Try to play your baby's favourite lullaby continuously, so when he awakens he can resettle himself to the familiar sleep-inducing sound of the lullabies.

4. Place your baby in a comfortable crib or bed. Especially in cold weather, you can have a flannel sheets or a warm towel placed on the sheets to provide them heat, and remove it before you put your baby on the warmed sheets.

5. Lessen physical discomforts of your baby. Free your baby's room from dust because they are known to be the common cause of babies' stuffy noses and consequent night-waking. Babies need to clear their nose to breathe. Although soon, they will learn to breathe alternatively through their mouth if their nose is blocked.

6. Most babies are disturbed by wet nappies at night, some are not. If the baby sleeps through wet nappies, there is no need to awaken him for a change except if your baby is experiencing nappy rash. For a continuous sleep, change the nappy just before a feeding, as baby is comfortable to fall asleep during or after feeding.

If your baby is still waking, bear in mind that his age may have to do with how he settles. An important thing to remember is that your baby's sleep habits are more a reflections of your baby's temper rather than your strategies of night-time parenting. Always remember that some parents usually exaggerate how long their baby sleeps, as if this would make other people say that you're a good parent, which it isn't.

Sleep Training, Three Important Steps

Are you exhausted from trying to rock or jiggle your baby to sleep? Only to have them wake the minute you lay them down. Parents are told that you can't spoil a newborn. This depends on your definition of the word spoil. I believe parents are constantly training their babies whether they realize it or not. It is possible to teach your newborn baby to fall asleep easily on their own with very little help from Mom and Dad.

As a certified infant specialist I am called on to help exhausted parents solve their baby's sleep issues. Many times these babies are 3 months of age or older. Most infant sleep issues could be easily avoided if parents understood the three necessary steps a baby passes through on their way to a sound sleep.

The most important thing you can do to help your baby learn healthy sleep habits is to lay them down while sleepy but awake. Rocking and holding your baby to sleep is something that even a newborn will quickly get used to. You are teaching them that they need this to be able to fall asleep. It is much better to reserve holding and rocking for when your baby is awake and alert.

There are three very definite stages that a baby passes through on the way to sleep. Understanding and recognizing these stages is critical in the success of sleep training your child.

1. The Wiggle Waggle Squirm Stage: This is the point where your baby is still awake and possibly fussy. They may grunt, squirm and fight the swaddle. Many parents tell me their baby hates the swaddle because they seem to fight it. This is actually a normal part of the learned process of falling asleep. This stage will last longer if you choose not to swaddle, as baby will startle and flail. The result will be a baby who takes longer to pass through the first stage of this process. Allow your baby at least 10 to 15 minutes to settle and move on to step two. Make sure that you have white noise playing loudly nearby. The white noise allows the babies nervous system to calm down and relax. If your baby is crying the white noise should be as loud as baby's cries.

2. The Five-Mile Stare: Once baby has passed through the fussy stage, they will get very still and stare into the distance. I call this the five-mile stare. Baby may lay quietly, looking into space for up to 15 minutes. If a noise startles baby when they are in this stage, they will most likely move back to stage one and squirm and fuss for a bit. It is very important that you do not pick baby up at this point. As long as they are not crying loudly for more than five minutes allow them to cycle back through to the five-mile stare. You can jiggle the baby in their swaddle and loudly shush in their ear, but try not to pick them up. This is a crucial step in baby learning to self soothe.

3. Sweet Sleep: Babies eyelids will begin to slowly close. They may yawn or slowly open and close their eyes several times. This is a sure sign that your baby is well on the way to sleeping peacefully.

Most parents do not realize that falling asleep on their own is a learned behavior. It is a very important and necessary skill that can be taught from the earliest days home from the hospital. Laying baby down while sleepy but awake and allowing them to fall asleep naturally is the most important first step. Understanding the normal stages that a baby passes through on their way to a deep sleep will help you be successful in sleep training your new baby.

The Effects of Sleep Training

With baby sleep training experts, doctors and parents all giving out advice on getting your baby to sleep with sexy headlines such as make your baby sleep from 7pm-7am it is no wonder many people are listening in. This training goes against our instincts and as you may have noticed feels horrible to sit through. I believe these beginnings in life are the most crucial and sleep training is destroying valuable bonds, relationships and trust.

When a baby cries it is calling for attention. Crying indicates that the baby is uncomfortable (wet, hot, cold), hungry, wind pain, scared or tired. A biological instinct in humans is to respond to this crying to ensure we address that need. It is the reason we can not stand a baby crying and why there is an urge to help. A baby will cry for a these reasons. If you solve these problems they will stop crying.

Overtired - Rock them off to sleep in your arms in a dark room.

➢ Wet Diaper/Nappy
➢ Cold or Hot
➢ Wind Pain
➢ Teething
➢ Headache, Fever or Illness

Not all problems above can just be solved quickly but at least comforting will help or you may be able to get something to soothe them. Also regardless of whether you just changed a diaper, check again! A baby comes into this world knowing that it has a mother and close family (including father) to look after and care for it. It doesn't know much else about the world as it has much to learn from you. So when they are placed in a quiet, dark room and are either scared or uncomfortable and they cried out for help and nobody came. They kept crying more and more and still nobody came. What does this teach them?

That when they are alone and scared or need help, no one is there to for them and they are in this world alone. When you see a world of people not caring about others do you think it might have stemmed from others not caring about them when they were first born? So when your baby is crying, comfort them, go in and ensure they are ok. It will result in getting up more, but in the long term they will self settle easier and be a more confident child knowing that if they do need help, you are there.

Sleep Training, Birth to 6 Months

Last night I spoke with the friend of mine who has 3-month-old. With complete respect, she sounded tired. She wanted answers. She was ready and willing to do anything if only to help her baby learn to sleep.

Had it been 3 months ago, when my LO was the age of hers, we probably would have just wept on the phone together, helpless. Her snapshot of all she had tried, heard, and read, resembled my efforts just the blink-of-an-eye ago.

She had a friend who told her she had successfully sleep trained her baby at 4 weeks old. She had read Baby Wise, The Baby Whisperer, and a host of other baby sleep training books. Not only that, but she has a Masters Degree in Early Childhood Education. As a teacher myself, I could completely relate to her desperation- by the book, she was trying everything she could to help her child, but on paper, nothing was working.

When will everyone get those much needed Z's again?

I remember trying to sleep train my LO around the same time that her friend claims to have had success. With a background in Applied Behavior Analysis, I thought this would be simple. I knew not to reinforce the behavior (crying) by going into the room, and I knew that intermittent reinforcement (going into the room sometimes, and not others) was even worse than going in every time.

"Blood curdling screams." My friend used that term last night too. That's what I heard when I tried to sleep train so young. Internally, I imagined throwing my fist through a wall.

I couldn't handle it. I remember one day after a valiant attempt at nap-time sleep training running into the nursery, sweeping my baby girl up, and just crying- holding her, crying, and promising her I'd never leave her again. (The behaviorists out there will probably shudder at that reinforcement.)

The thing that the books don't tell you is that every child is different. As much as we want to compartmentalize learning, (and we do- look at our school systems,) it's just not reality. My mom swears I slept through the night at 3 months, never cried, and went straight from the breast to a cup. Does that mean my child will do those things? No. Does that mean my mom's memory might be slightly tainted? Maybe just a little.

Here's what my sleep training time line looks like, (roughly, I'm already having difficulty remembering), from birth to 6 months:

- Birth to 6 weeks- Lots of sleeping during the day, numerous unsuccessful attempts to wake my child for daytime fun, and inconsolable crying from about 6PM - 2AM.

What helped? Walking around the house holding my baby *sometimes* made her crying a little more subdued. Sitting with her was not an option, rocking her in a rocking chair didn't help, and she didn't care if the lighting was low- (one time I actually tripped over a dog toy trying to calm her with the lights off at 1 AM, but miraculously she remained safe in my arms.)

- 6-10 weeks- Noted improvement in nighttime sleep, still waking every 3 hours at night to eat. The only way to get her to go to sleep though, (and this was true from birth,) was to put her in a vibrating bouncy seat, bounce her with one foot, and play the guitar for her. We wanted very much to put her bouncy seat in her crib and call it a night, but it just wasn't safe. My husband would stay in the living room with her while I got a few winks in the bed; then when she stirred to eat, I would pick her up, bring her to her room, nurse her, and put her in the crib. Most naps were in the car or in the bouncy seat.

- 10-14 weeks- More of the same, with interspersed attempts at sleep training. One time I was at my parents' house attempting to put my LO down for a nap. "We fully support you," my mom told me as we listened to the screams outside the door. Her face told a completely different story though- she longed for me to stop torturing my child! Still waking every 3 hours at night to eat.

- 14 weeks to 5 ½ months- I believe it was around this point that we said, "She's got to go down in her crib at night." To transition her, when we saw her start to fall asleep in her bouncer, we moved her to the crib. With the lights down low, we took 15-minute shifts of playing the guitar to a screaming baby. After a little over an hour, our child was asleep, and we never went back to sleeping in the bouncy chair. As for naps, I feared I was indeed torturing my child, and I continued to rock her in my arms at the expense of my back. Still waking every 3 hours (and often more often) at night to eat.

- 5 ½ - 6 ½ months- This was when we upgraded to the video baby monitor. My back simply could not handle the weight of my 97th percentile baby every time she needed to sleep. By this time we were good at recognizing the signs that she was sleepy- eye rubbing, yawning, fussiness, and after reading her a book or 2 and putting on a playlist of classical music, I began putting her down for nap-time and bedtime without turning back.

I also recently spoke with the doctor's office about her night-waking. "97th percentile? She's definitely getting all the food she needs. Let her cry herself back to sleep when she wakes at night, and she'll learn to get out of that habit."

It wasn't easy. When she woke the first time and I didn't go in it was an hour-and-a-half before she was sleeping again. But between the monitor, her age, and the support of my husband and the doctor's office, I was able to do it.

Now she cries for about 10 minutes after sleeping for 6 hours, goes back to sleep, and wants to nurse after a good 8-9 hours of sleep. (She even goes back down after this, sleeping in total at night for 11-12 hours.)

So it does get better, But I really do believe that every child is different. You have to do what's best for your child, yourself, and your family. And for people who love to apply learned information, this can be very frustrating. Being a mother brings the concept of trusting yourself to a whole new level. "It's humbling," my friend said last night, and I couldn't agree more.

Baby Sleep Training - How to Mimic the Feeling of the Womb

For the entire beginning of their lives, babies are accustomed to one environment: the womb. It can be very jarring to come into a new world with so much new stimuli, and it can cause a feeling of insecurity in baby. The best way to help baby sleep more soundly, make the transition, and feel safe is to mimic some of the feelings of the womb.

Characteristics of The Womb

So what does the womb have that your house doesn't? Let's think about the environment baby is familiar with:

Lots of white noise - he's used to a very loud environment, what with the outside noises mixing with the sounds of the body's machinery

Cramped quarters - he's used to existing in a very small space, where everything is close together

Feeling supported - he's used to being touched and supported on the sides and bottom of the womb, which creates a sense of comfort from being touched

Fetal position - he's accustomed to laying in the fetal position, with the arms and legs drawn up and close to the body

As you read this, birth might seem to come as a relief. To us, the womb doesn't seem very comfortable, but to baby, it's home. You can ease the transition and help baby sleep by mimicking some of these qualities

Why Does This Feeling Help Baby Sleep? We've already talked about this, but it's important enough to say again. Babies, even in the womb, are extremely sensitive to emotions and feelings. Just like you, baby doesn't sleep well if she's not relaxed and feeling safe.

It comes as a domino effect: if baby is anxious or in some other way emotionally upset, she can't relax. When she can't relax, and you put her to bed and leave, she gets more upset, which makes it take even longer to relax. Until she relaxes, she can't fall asleep, and crying ensues.

Swaddle Baby

Swaddling baby can help her relax and settle down because it mimics the close quarters of the womb. Babies can be unsettled by the free use of their arms and legs after birth, a feeling they didn't have in the womb. Additionally, babies tend to jerk a bit upon falling asleep and can wake themselves up or become startled by these natural movements.

Swaddling baby all the time is fine for the first month of life; after that, baby needs access to her arms and legs to develop properly.

However, you can still swaddle baby for naps and nighttime to help her sleep.

So what is Swaddling?

Swaddling is wrapping baby tightly in a blanket to mimic the feeling of the womb. Swaddling reminds baby of the safety and compact feeling of the womb.

How to swaddle Baby

Lay a baby blanket on the floor and fold one corner into the center about 6 inches

Lay baby on her back on the blanket, with her head at the folded-down corner. The head should be off the blanket so it's free

Take the corner near baby's left hand and pull it across baby to the right, securing it underneath baby

Fold up the bottom of the blanket towards baby's chin, enclosing baby's feet

Take the corner near baby's right hand and pull it across baby to the left, securing it underneath baby

Important Tips

Swaddle baby when she is full, clean, and dry. Swaddling is meant to be a comfortable, comforting experience for baby, and if she is in some way unsettled, she will associate bad memories with swaddling.

Don't swaddle baby when it is very hot. Keep baby from overheating by not swaddling when it is very hot outside or when baby is in a warm room. This is especially important when baby is going to sleep, as overheating is a risk factor for SIDS.

Listen to baby so you know when she wants out. Baby will kick or squirm when she wants to be free, so pay attention for these actions. Let baby out if you know she is uncomfortable, or the feeling can cause distress and keep baby from relaxing.

Don't swaddle baby constantly after the age of one month. She needs access to her limbs in order to develop correctly.

Action Items:

> ➢ Find or buy a baby blanket
> ➢ Practice swaddling a doll before attempting it on your live, squirming baby
> ➢ Pay attention to baby's reaction to being swaddled and adjust if necessary
> ➢ Strategies for Mimicking the Womb Bathe baby in a bucket

There are a host of products available that offer an alternative to a mini-adult-like bath. Baths can be a pivotal relaxation tool each day to help baby sleep, mostly because being immersed in water reminds them of being in the womb.

Naturally, you can see that how you bathe baby becomes an important part of helping baby calm down and fall asleep. Babies feel most comfortable in the fetal position, and a bucket provides this capability. It supports baby's weight and allows her to be touched on the sides and the bottom of the bucket, again reminding her of the womb.

A bucket is a natural choice for a bath because it almost forces baby into the fetal position. This combined with warm water and the tightness of baby touching the sides and bottom of the bucket work together to recreate the feeling of the womb. As opposed to a bucket, a mini-adult-like bath gives baby the feeling of swimming, like in the womb, but makes her feel a bit lost, with nothing to control her arms and legs from floating around.

I know, it seems almost cruel to put your baby in a bucket, right? Think outside the box! It only seems strange because not many people do it...in the United States, that is. Bathing baby in a bucket is a popular form of baby care in Europe and is accepted as helping to calm and reassure babies in this big new world.

Quick tip: there's no need to go buy an expensive baby bathing bucket, though you certainly can. Use what you have at home, but be sure to choose a bucket you have not used with harsh chemicals. Think of a bucket used to build sand castles, perhaps. If possible, find a bucket with flexible sides, so that baby is supported softly and without any sharp edges or seams.

Action Items:

- ➢ Find a baby-sized bucket in the house and thoroughly clean it, or purchase a new one
- ➢ Confirm that the bucket is flexible, smooth, and won't tip over when baby is inside
- ➢ Test a bath to see if baby likes the feeling of a bucket better than a traditional baby bath
- ➢ Sway and Shush Your Baby To Sleep

When a mother moves around doing daily tasks, a baby in the womb is naturally swung gently from side to side. This swaying motion becomes familiar and comforting, so parents can try using this as a means of calming baby before sleep. Remember, this isn't the kind of thing that you want to do every time that baby wakes up, or you will have to repeatedly get up in the middle of the night.

Instead, this is what you want to do to help settle baby down so that she can fall asleep on her own. When swaying baby, be gentle and consistent. She should fall into a sort of rhythm that helps calm her.

Swaying shouldn't be fast or exciting, as it's meant to relax baby. Sway her too fast and she'll think it's playtime instead.

Shushing is another technique that mimics the womb. This is similar to the sounds that baby hears in the womb and can also be quieting. As with swaying, shushing should be gentle and rhythmic. It should be smooth and mimic the pattern of baby's breathing - one "shush" per exhale.

Shushing should be soft, not harsh; avoid the sound a teacher makes when quieting her classroom. Instead, use shushing as a sort of white noise, meant to calm baby without her ever even realizing it.

Action Items:

> ➢ Sing a song in your head while you sway or shush to help create a slow rhythm
> ➢ Try different speeds and voice levels to find out what quiets baby best
> ➢ Wear Baby

Another solution that feels similar to the womb is wearing baby in a sling, wrap, or pouch. This has benefits for you, because it allows you to be close to baby while keeping your hands free, and it makes baby feel protected, safe, and comfortable.

Wearing baby helps keep baby warm, lets her hear your heartbeat, and builds a close relationship that is fostered through personal contact. Listed here are a few options for wearing baby, but it's up to you to decide which solution is best and most comfortable for you and baby:

Wrap - wraps are long pieces of fabric tied to the wearer in various positions. Baby folds up inside it and it is very versatile. This is best for small babies; larger children will have trouble fitting, and it could be uncomfortable for the wearer.

Mei Tai - an Asian-inspired carrier with more structure than a wrap. It can be worn on the front, back, or hip, depending on comfort and baby's size. This is a viable option for larger or older babies.

Adjustable pouch - a pouch is a circle of fabric tied onto the wearer's front that holds the baby into the wearer's chest. It is similar to a Mei Tai and is also good for babies of all sizes.

Action Items:

- ➤ Evaluate your needs and baby's size to determine which style is right for you
- ➤ Practice tying on a wrap, sling or pouch with a doll prior to working with baby
- ➤ Adjust the fit as necessary - if baby seems uncomfortable, evaluate her fit to see if anything is rubbing or pinching. Try putting baby in while sitting down to see if this helps
- ➤ Consider different options as baby grows and your activities change. Some ways to wear baby are more appropriate for some types of activities than others

CHAPTER TWO
Baby Sleep Techniques

If you are a new parent, you probably have been looking for baby sleep techniques in order to help your infant snooze better at night. You are not alone! Many new parents are suffering from sleep deprivation and this usually continues until the child is about a year old, sometimes longer. But by following these simple tips you will be sure to see the black circles under your eyes quickly disappear and you'll feel more refreshed and energized in no time.

The most important of all baby sleep techniques is to get your baby on a schedule as quickly as possible, and definitely by eight weeks old. The general rule of thumb is to follow the feeding, changing, playtime and nap time pattern throughout the day so that your infant gets to know the routine and begins to anticipate what comes next in the pattern. In addition to the daytime schedule, build a nighttime schedule as well. It could be as simple as a bath followed by a bottle, then you put your babe down in the crib for the evening. Just follow the same steps each night and the little one will gradually begin to realize that after the bath comes a bottle and then it is time for sleep.

Some baby sleep techniques will work for other babies but may not work for yours. However, I highly recommend swaddling your baby before bed at least during the first three months. It tends to work wonders for infants who crave the snugness and coziness that they were used to in the womb. Always put your child to sleep on his or her back, per the American Association of Pediatrics' guidelines for preventing sudden infant death syndrome or SIDS. They also recommend that babies use a pacifier at night as that seems to lower the risk of SIDS as well.

How to Solve Baby Sleep Problems

Babies are instinctive creatures, and they are made to sense what they need when they need it. Attempting to make your baby learn something he or she is not ready for is not healthy in any way physically, mentally, and may even lead to future problems. It will also be unsuccessful and ineffective. Let's look at some of the baby sleep problems.

Babies need warmth, comfort, and a sense of trust that they will be taken care of and responded to when needed. This applies to eating and sleeping also. One of the biggest, most harmful mistakes of modern times is that of the cry it out method.

Babies cannot talk or tell anyone what they need this is why they cry. It is an alert that they do need something. Granted, many babies seem to be easier to deal with when it comes to sleep, and others seem almost intent on keeping everyone awake.

It will have to be accepted as a new parent that you will lose sleep. You can make this issue more comfortable to deal with for both you and baby. Too many sleepless nights will lead to intense stress and frustration for the parent; this will also affect baby.

It is important to eliminate the sleep training method now. This is a ridiculous and cruel answer, and actually creates more problems and heartache for parent and child alike.

You should also consider that later on, you will miss your child being a baby, and the smells and cuddling that are a part of this special time. Do you want to look back and regret the way you handled your helpless baby? Babies cry because they need something; we should not ignore this need.

A baby needs to feel trust, and comfort in the fact that his needs will be met when he needs them to be. When this does not occur, especially repeatedly, the baby will grow into a child and then adult who may not trust anyone. In addition, this may lead to pathology.

Some babies prefer being in their own room in their crib. Others need to feel that the parent is very near this is where a bassinet can be used, as it is placed beside the bed. Rocking, patting, and swaddling are frequently surefire methods for mom to use to comfort and reassure baby. Self-soothing tips can be tried as well; however, this does not mean baby is to be left alone to cry, nor should he be hovered over the whole night unless he is ill.

Keeping baby busy with games, singing and swinging etc. In the daytime will often give baby a restful evening. Do not give up; utilizing various ideas and testing out personal preferences can guide you and your baby to resolving baby sleep problems. This is a precious time; do not allow it to lead to future problems for your child and regret for yourself. These are moments that can never be recaptured.

Baby Sleeping Facts

All people need sleep. Sleeping is important because it gives individuals the time for the body to recuperate and regenerate. Adults need a 6 to 8 hours of sleep to relax, while babies need a complete 8 hours of sleep and naps in between. Sleeping has a lot use in a human's life and it includes cell regeneration and condition the nervous system and overall helps in the development of our body, mind and health. Babies need sleep to develop muscles, extremities, skeletal structure, brain and other organs. In addition, sleep helps the body regenerate fingernails, toenails, hair and skin. Sleep stimulates your baby's growth and development and when this is achieved, your baby can reach a healthy life.

Choosing The Right Bed

It is always ideal to prepare a safe sleeping environment for your baby before he arrives at home. You can purchase a cute crib and necessary sheets from stores. Baby retail outlets personnel can advise you about the best type of bedding for your baby. In order to put your baby in a good night sleep, the bed or crib is one that feels just right. It is very essential that your baby have a comfortable bed and a calm environment to promote sleep.

The baby's bed should not necessarily be cozy, but it should provide security for them to get a good night sleep. The sheets should be comfortable and soft for your baby's delicate skin. A sheet that is rough or even too fluffy diminishes you baby's comfort thus, it causes sleep interruption. The bed should also be pleasant for your baby's eyes. There is a wide selection of colourful designs and fabrics in the market today that choosing a good quality bedding a fun and easy task for parents.

Sleeping With Your Baby

Advantages

The main advantage in sleeping with your baby is the increased bonding time. It is convenient for you because it is easy to have your baby on your side especially when you are breastfeeding and being near is comforting for your baby. According to research, babies who sleep next to their mothers have less interrupted sleep and cry less. Co-sleeping provides your baby warmth, sound, scent, touches and other sensory stimuli that make your baby respond in a positive way. Sleeping with your baby is very safe and beneficial. However, it depends upon the situation. If the parents smoke or take illegal drugs, sleeping with your baby is risky.

Disadvantages

Not sleeping with your baby predisposes him to potential risks such as accidental falls and aspiration from neglected bottle feeding. In addition, it is always ideal to use a firm but comfortable mattress, and limit the use of pillow and blankets. This could also be hard for your relationship because you might be near with your baby but less so with your partner since you may be putting or using the baby as a gap between you and your partner. Sleeping with your baby requires certain precautions be taken to assure baby safety.

Why Baby Sleep Is So Important

Sleep...it's something that we all need. It is crucial for parents, babies, toddlers and well, everyone! Unfortunately many of us don't get enough of it - our babies included.

We all need sufficient amounts of sleep in order to function properly, and it is particularly important in the development of these babies and young children. It is well known that sleep deprived adults have difficulty focusing and functioning and may suffer mental and physical health problems in the long-term. So too, one cannot expect an exhausted little baby to function effectively when sleep deprived either!

Sleep is essential for physical and mental rejuvenation, a functioning immune system, healthy growth, and emotional well being. Without enough sleep, your baby will become fretful, irritable and inconsolable. And to make matters worse, sleep-deprivation in early infancy will further interfere with their longer-term capacity for deep, restful sleep.

Babies and children who don't get enough sleep are often unjustly labeled 'fussy' and 'temperamental', when in reality they are simply too exhausted to function properly. It goes without saying that babies who suffer from this poor quality of sleep often have parents who are also exhausted, and thereby unable to enjoy, care for and nurture their children as they would like.

According to a recent study by the National Sleep Association, more than 70% of infants and toddlers have some type of sleep problem.

If not treated, more than 50% of babies who suffer from sleep problems will continue to experience problems through pre-school and school-age.

An insufficient amount of sleep in babies and children is detrimental to health, behavior, mood, attention, memory and learning ability.

Some parents think that they have irritable, inconsolable babies. "My baby cries all day even when he's awake...of COURSE he's difficult!" Fussy - yes. Chronically irritable - no. Some babies may be a bit more sensitive and temperamental, but babies who are crying so much are doing so for a reason. Assuming there are no medical complications and that a baby is not in pain, your baby may be crying during the day simply because he's tired! Even if he catches random cat naps here and there, it won't solve the overall sleep deprivation that is so crucial to his well being.

So first things first. If you think your baby isn't getting the sufficient amount of sleep to function properly and be well rested, it's time to do something about it. Take note of his daily behavior and ask yourself some questions:

> How many naps does he take daily?
> How long are these naps?
> How long does he stay awake between naps?
> How much sleep is he getting at night?

After figuring out your baby's basic patterns, you may want to reconfigure certain aspects of his daily sleep in order to insure your baby is well-rested and happy.

Sleep Training Your Baby: 7 Tips for Success

The human brain runs on sleep. The American Academy of Sleep Medicine recommends that infants aged 4-12 months get between 12-16 hours of sleep during each 24-hour period (including naps) to reap the most health benefits. Children ages 1-2 years need 11-14 hours, and those ages 3-5 need 10-13 hours a day.

Not catching enough Zzz's can have numerous consequences for babies and parents. Indeed, the American Academy of Pediatrics (AAP) has linked frequent night wakings to postpartum depression in moms, future childhood obesity, behavioral problems, and more. Marc Weissbluth, M.D., the author of Healthy Sleep Habits, Happy Child, adds that babies who don't get enough consolidated REM sleep have shorter attention spans, so they don't learn as well. They also release more of the stress hormone cortisol, setting them up for frequent night wakings and stunted naps.

The key to combating these negative consequences? Starting an effective sleep-training method that works for your child. If necessary, talk to your pediatrician to rule out any underlying medical condition (such as GERD, sleep apnea, or allergies) that may be keeping your child awake at night. Then make sure you and your partner are on the same page, and follow these tips for sleep training your baby.

1. Keep a Sleep Log

Keeping a log can help you notice patterns in your baby's sleep schedule. Start by tracking days and nights for one week, then use the data to figure out their ideal bedtime. You might say, "Oh, she's always fussy at 7 p.m.—that's probably when I should be putting her down." A log might also let you see that your infant isn't crying as often as you thought; five minutes of fussing can feel like 50 minutes at 2 a.m.

2. Create a Bedtime Routine

Each night, perform bedtime rituals that will ease your baby's mind and prepare their body for sleep. Include soothing techniques such as bathing, reading, or singing lullabies. Keep anything stimulating like tickling, watching TV, or playing with electronic toys out of the equation. Following a consistent routine lets your baby know it's time for bed, and it also develops their internal clock.

3. Pick an Effective Start Date

There's never a perfect time to start sleep training, but avoid scheduling it around major events in your baby's life (time changes, a new nanny, teething, a different bedroom, etc.) Most parents begin on Friday to take advantage of the upcoming weekend and some use vacation days so they won't have to worry about sleep deprivation at work. And remember: You'll always be more successful if your baby has been napping well.

4. Set the Nursery Scene

When it comes to sleep training your baby, the environment is extremely important. Keep the room cool and comfortable, preferably between 65 and 70 degrees. If your baby's room gets a lot of light and she has trouble with naps and early wake-ups consider installing room-darkening shades.

5. Choose a Sleep-Training Technique

Effective sleep-training tactics vary by family and child. Here are a few popular options to consider.

Fading Method: With this method, parents help their baby fall asleep with soothing techniques (feeding, rocking, talking, etc.) Your baby will naturally require less comfort over time, so you can gradually "fade out" of their bedtime routine.

Ferber Method: Parents check on their crying child at gradually increasing time intervals, which promotes self-soothing and independent sleeping.

Pick-Up/Put-Down Method: Parents pick up their baby when they cry or fuss, then put them down after they're comforted, repeating until they fall asleep.

Cry It Out Method: After their bedtime routine, babies are left to "cry it out" until they fall asleep independently.

Chair Method: Mom or Dad sits next to the crib in a chair until the baby falls asleep, trying not to soothe if they get fussy. They gradually move the chair further from the crib each night, until they're outside of the room and out of view.

6. Ditch the Sleep Crutches

No matter which sleep-training method you choose, it's important to stop sleep crutches (like rocking, singing, or nursing to sleep) when your infant is older than 3 or 4 months, says Kim West, author of Good Night, Sleep Tight: The Sleep Lady's Gentle Guide to Helping Your Baby Go to Sleep. "These are not negative or bad behaviors," says West, "but they become a problem when they're so closely linked in the child's mind with slumber that he cannot drift off without them." Continuing with these sleep crutches will mean every time your baby wakes up, they'll need you to rock, sing, or nurse them but your goal is actually to teach them to self-soothe and put themself back to sleep.

7. Stay Consistent

One of the biggest mistakes parents make, no matter what sleep-training method they use, is being inconsistent. At some point, your little one will cry for you in the middle of the night even if you think you've all made it over the sleep-training hump. Check on them to make sure all is well; just be sure not to restart an old sleep crutch during this check. After that, try comforting them from outside the door, if you can. If you regress due to illness or travel, get back on the training wagon as soon as possible. Otherwise you risk sabotaging the weeks of hard work you've already put in.

Bedtime Routines

You can start a bedtime routine as early as you like in your baby's life. It is a way of indicating the difference between night and day.

How to do it

Start the bedtime routine 30-40 minutes before you would like your baby or child to go to sleep.

The bedtime routine should be relaxing and predictable with the same things happening every night at about the same time.

The routine could include a bath or nappy change, a massage, putting on night clothes, a breastfeed or a warm drink, teeth cleaning, a story, a lullaby, relaxing music.

Turn off all screens (TVs, computers, tablets, phones) at least 30 minutes before bedtime. Looking at screens just before bedtime can stop children from sleeping well.

Once ready for bed, your baby or child should not return to main living area.

The bedtime routine should finish in the bedroom with the last part of the routine (eg a story or a lullaby) happening with your baby or child in bed.

Do look out for signs that your child is sleepy when deciding on a good bedtime, for example:

Do

> Being less active,
> Slower movements,
> Making fewer noises,
> Suckling more slowly and gently,
> Being quieter and calmer,
> Seeming less interested in surroundings,
> Eyes focussing less,
> Eyelids drooping.

Don't

Don't include things in the bedtime routine that you won't be happy to repeat every evening.

Don't make a bath part of your child's bedtime routine if it is not practical for your child to have a bath every night.

Encouraging independent settling in babies

You can start trying to encourage independent settling for naps and night time sleeps as early as you like in your baby's life. Some of these ideas may be easier to try when your baby is a bit older - for example, when they don't always fall asleep while feeding.

How to do it

Learn to tell when your baby is sleepy.

Put your baby down to sleep when he or she is drowsy but awake.

Avoid feeding or cuddling your baby to sleep.

Try warming the bed before putting your baby down to sleep.

Put something that smells of you in bed with your baby. Choose something that can't cover your baby's head or mouth.

Give your baby a toy or blanket to hold while feeding that they take to bed with them.

Consider swaddling your baby. Your Health Visitor can give you information about how to do this safely.

Make night time boring by keeping the room dark and talking quietly and as little as possible.

White noise, lullabies and calming music can help a baby to settle.

Do

Do continue to feed your baby on demand day and night. Night time feeds are important for a baby's growth and for breast milk production.

Do keep your baby in the same room as you, day and night, for at least the first six months.

Do look out for signs that your child is sleepy:

> ➤ Decreased activity,
> ➤ Slower movements,
> ➤ Making fewer noises,
> ➤ Suckling more slowly and gently,
> ➤ Being quieter and calmer,
> ➤ Seeming less interested in
> ➤ Surroundings,
> ➤ Eyes focussing less,
> ➤ Eyelids drooping.

Don't

Don't worry if your newborn baby always falls asleep while feeding – as they get older it will be easier to put them down when they are drowsy but awake.

Don't feel that you have to do this if you are happy cuddling and feeding your baby to sleep. You can encourage independent sleep later if you want to.

Pick up, put Down

This is a sleep training technique for a baby or toddler who does not settle to sleep well or who wakes frequently during the night. It involves comforting the baby but not feeding them every time they wake up. It can be very frustrating and difficult for parents but is usually effective quickly.

How to do it

Have a consistent, positive bedtime routine.

Put your baby to bed when they are drowsy but awake.

If your baby cries, pick them up and say, "shh, I'm here, it's OK."

Once you you have reassured them, and they are still awake, put them down.

If they cry once they are down, pick them up and reassure them again, then put them down and leave the room.

Whenever they cry, go back in, pick them up and reassure them.

As soon as the crying stops, put them down and leave the room.

If they struggle and fight you, say, "shh, I'm here" and put them straight back down.

With an older child, don't automatically pick them up, but say reassuring words and offer to pick them up if that is what they want.

Repeat this whenever the baby or child wakes during the night or after night feeds.

If you are feeding your baby during the night when using this technique, feed your baby at planned times in a particular chair. See the information about reducing night feeds.

Do

> ➢ Do be prepared for this to take a long time. Some babies take up to three hours to settle when beginning this technique.
> ➢ Do get support from a partner, relative or friend.
> ➢ Do expect to have backache .
> ➢ Do tell your baby, "It's ok, I love you, you can do this, you are ok, it's ok to be upset, you can do it." This will help you to stay calm.
> ➢ Do be prepared to feel cross and frustrated.

Don't

> ➢ Don't use this technique with babies younger than three months old.
> ➢ Don't stop responding to your baby's requests for night feeds until they are at least six months old.
> ➢ Don't be surprised if there are some peaks of crying when you are using this technique.

Gradual Retreat

This technique is a way of helping a baby or child get used to going to sleep without their parent or carer in the room. It can be useful for children who need to be fed or cuddled to sleep. It is a gentle technique which is unlikely to cause distress to the child or parent. It may take some weeks to be effective.

It is useful for toddlers and children who do not need to feed at night and who are old enough to understand that their parent is still in the room when they are not touching.

How to do it

- ➢ Have a consistent, positive bedtime routine.
- ➢ Say goodnight and sit on a chair or cushion next to the bed.
- ➢ If they cry, gently put your hand on them. Avoid eye contact.
- ➢ When the crying stops, go back and sit on the chair or cushion.
- ➢ Repeat every time they cry and stay in the room until they are asleep.
- ➢ Return and repeat whenever your child wakes up during the night.
- ➢ Each night, move the chair or cushion slightly further away from the bed. If your child is upset by this, bring it back to the last night's position.
- ➢ Once the chair is outside the room, your child is ready to go to sleep by themselves.

Gradual Retreat

Do

- ➢ Do move the chair or cushion back several times during one bedtime if it is going well.
- ➢ Do go at your child's pace.

Don't

Don't be surprised if it takes several weeks until your baby or child goes to sleep happily on their own using this technique.

The Kissing Game

This is a gentle sleep training technique for helping a toddler or older child to get used to going to sleep without their parent in the room with them. It is similar to Gradual Retreat.

How to do it:

➢ Have a consistent, positive bedtime routine.
➢ Put your baby or child to bed when they are drowsy but awake and kiss them goodnight.
➢ Promise to return in a few moments to give them another kiss.
➢ Return almost immediately to give a kiss.
➢ Take a few steps to the door, then return immediately to give a kiss.
➢ Promise to return in a few moments to give them another kiss.
➢ Put something away or do something in the room then give them a kiss.
➢ As long as the child stays in bed, keep returning to give more kisses.
➢ Do something outside their room and return to give kisses.
➢ If the child gets out of bed, say, "back into bed and I'll give you a kiss".
➢ Keep returning frequently to give kisses until they are asleep.
➢ Repeat every time the child wakes during the night.

Do

➢ Do be prepared for this to take a long time when you first start – it may take three hours and 300 kisses until your child falls asleep.
➢ Do substitute strokes and pats for kisses if your baby is in a cot and you can't reach in to kiss them.

Don't

Don't try this with a baby younger than 12 months old

This is a sleep training technique for a baby aged over six months or a toddler who does not settle to sleep well or who wakes frequently during the night. It involves comforting the baby but not picking them up or feeding them. It involves listening to some minutes of crying which may be distressing for parents. It is usually effective quickly.

How to do it

> ➤ Have a consistent, positive bedtime routine.
> ➤ Put your baby down to sleep when they are drowsy but awake.
> ➤ Say "goodnight" quietly and leave the room.
> ➤ If your baby cries, wait two minutes, go back and say "go to sleep, I'm here, it's OK" but don't lift them up.
> ➤ Leave the room again.
> ➤ If your baby cries again, wait three minutes, go back in and say "go to sleep, I'm here, OK" but don't lift them.
> ➤ Leave the room again.
> ➤ Repeat as many times as necessary increasing waiting time to a maximum of 10 minutes.
> ➤ If your baby stands up, place your hands on their body and quietly encourage them to lie down each time. Praise them when they lie down.
> ➤ If your child gets out of bed, return them to the bed without speaking and without eye contact every time they get out.
> ➤ If your baby vomits from crying and you wish to persevere with controlled crying, change their clothes and sheets quietly without eye contact and leave the room again.
> ➤ If your child wrecks their room, leave the mess. Don't tidy up until the sleep training is complete.
> ➤ Be consistent – it may take more than an hour before your baby or child goes to sleep. It may take a week before your baby goes to sleep without a fuss.
> ➤ Repeat the technique if your child wakes during the night

Do

> ➤ Do choose a week when you have no other plans.
> ➤ Do get a partner, friend or relative to support you.
> ➤ Do tell your neighbours.
> ➤ Do make sure your baby gets plenty of love and attention in the daytime.
> ➤ Do make sure that the bedroom is safe and warm.

Don't

> ➤ Don't use this technique if your baby is younger than six months.
> ➤ Don't use this technique until you are happy that your baby can go all night without a feed. You can discuss this with your Health Visitor.
> ➤ Don't use this technique if your baby or child is ill.
> ➤ Don't continue for more than two weeks if it doesn't work

Co-Sleeping

Many parents find that their baby settles easily to sleep if they share a bed for some or all of the night, or just some nights. This can make breastfeeding easier and mean fewer disturbances at night. Choosing to co-sleep when your baby is very young doesn't mean that they will never be able to sleep on their own.

How to do it

> ➤ Make sure your bed is safe for your baby and that they can't fall out, get covered by duvets, pillows, pets or siblings or get too hot.
> ➤ Make sure that your partner knows that your baby is in the bed.
> ➤ Learn how to breastfeed lying down. Your Health Visitor or breastfeeding group can show you how to do this comfortably.

- Read the information overleaf and in the UNICEF leaflet "Caring for Your Baby at Night" about safe co-sleeping.
- When you are ready to move your child out of your bed, you might find that this happens easily, or you might want to try some of the sleep training methods that your Health visitor can suggest.

Do

- Do look at the information on bedtime routines. This can still be useful when cosleeping.
- Do look at the information on establishing independent sleep in babies.

Don't

- Don't sleep with your baby on a sofa or water bed.
- Don't sleep with your baby in your bed if you or your partner smoke.
- Don't sleep with your baby in your bed if you or your partner have been drinking alcohol or are taking medications which make you sleepy.
- Don't sleep with your baby if you or your baby are ill or have a high temperature.
- Don't sleep with your baby if he or she is very small or was born prematurely.

Reducing Night Feeds

This can be useful for older babies and toddlers who wake frequently to feed at night. All babies develop at slightly different rates, but many babies can cope without feeding in the night from around six months onwards. Some babies stop asking for night feeds when they are younger than this.

How to do it

- ➤ Discuss with your Health Visitor or breastfeeding group your baby's readiness to sleep longer at night without feeding.
- ➤ If you are breastfeeding, reduce night feeds gradually to avoid developing blocked ducts or mastitis.
- ➤ First drop the feeds when you would prefer not to wake up. You might decide that you don't want to feed your baby between midnight and 5am, for example, but that you are happy to feed at other times.
- ➤ Offer your baby a cup of water when they ask to feed in the night. You might want to try "pick up, put down" at these times.
- ➤ If your baby is bottlefed, gradually dilute their night time milk with water and give it in a cup

Do

- ➤ Do breastfeed on demand day and night in the early months to establish a good milk supply.
- ➤ Do respond to your baby's cues to feed frequently in the evenings (sometimes called cluster feeding).
- ➤ Do give your baby clear signs when you are happy to feed at night – eg by picking them up and sitting in a particular chair.

Don't

- ➤ Don't reduce night feeds if your baby is struggling with weight gain.
- ➤ Don't wake your baby for a "dream feed" as this may encourage them to wake for feeds at night

CHAPTER THREE

Why Isn't My Baby Sleeping?

Y ou are a brand new parent and you've just brought that little bundle of joy home. You are eager to begin your journey as a loving and patient parent. And then you find that Baby doesn't always want to sleep when you do; in fact he appears to fight sleep. And once he goes to sleep he doesn't stay asleep.

Baby's Sleep Window

The first is that you may have missed your baby's sleep window. The "sleep window" is when the baby quiets and goes to sleep on his own. He is tired and knows it and is ready for sleep. If you miss this he will be over tired and will fight sleep. The remedy for this may be moving bedtime to an earlier time or a later time. If he's fighting sleep the earlier bedtime will help.

Too Much Sleep?

The second reason may be that your baby simply has slept too much during the day and isn't really tired. This is more likely to be something toddlers do, not newborns. For this problem you'll want to have a later bedtime for your baby.

Separation Anxiety

The third reason is that your baby might be going through separation anxiety and he simply misses you. This is more likely to happen with older babies though. If you think this is the problem you can go to him to reassure him from time to time.

Personality & Temperament

The fourth reason is this may simply be your baby's personality and temperament. Perceptive and social babies may fight sleep because they enjoy the stimulation of being awake and more interesting. They don't want to miss a moment of fun! I think this is why my grandson Emory is hard to get to sleep at night. My solution for this is to play with him until he goes to sleep on his own.

According to the research your baby may go through a sleep regression at 4 months. Babies don't have sleep cycles like adults do. We go between deep and light sleep but babies don't do that. At 4 months the brain matures and your baby's sleep changes to be more like yours. This is normal and healthy but also means that your baby is cycling between deep and light sleep and when awakening from light sleep will have a harder time going back to sleep. The changes that happen during this regression are permanent which is really a good thing. You do want that little brain to mature normally after all. Don't hesitate to call on other family members to help you so you don't become exhausted from lack of sleep yourself.

The following are some suggestions to help your baby fall asleep:

Swaddling and/or a Binkie

Swaddling sometimes helps your baby fall asleep as does a pacifier. Swaddling makes them feel safe and warm and if your baby likes the Binkie this will make him feel contented.

Rocking or a Swing

If you've been rocking your baby to sleep continue it. Keep doing whatever you've been doing to help your baby sleep. Another thing you can do is use a swing or a cradle; the motion of the swing or cradle is often soothing for them and sleep inducing.

Dream Feed

Then there is what is called the Dream Feed. This is where your baby is asleep and you give him a bottle. Don't pick him up or wake him, just put a bottle in his mouth and hold it until he is finished drinking. This will help your baby sleep longer so you can too.

Now, you can begin sleep training. This simply entails teaching your baby to fall asleep alone without rocking or eating. This means you'll wait until your baby is drowsy but still awake and then put him to bed. Hopefully, your baby will go on to sleep but it could take weeks to accomplish so this isn't a quick fix like rocking, and dream feed. This will take patience.

Now you know it is normal for your baby to fight sleep, why and what you can do about it! Other family members can help you with all of this so have patience and love and you'll all get through this.

Baby Sleep Tips When Teething

Many parents wonder if teething might have an impact at their baby's sleep. The teething often starts just when a baby starts to sleep through the night. This can be frustrating for many parents especially for new parents as they thought that all the tiring night has now ended but suddenly it comes back again. However it does not mean that everything your baby has achieved with independent sleeping has to go out of the window.

Teething can start at between four to six months old. However it might take awhile before the actual tooth appears.

Teething can take up to two years old of age and can lead to toddler night waking. Some babies have mild sign of teething such as drooling and chewing on everything, while other babies can have moderate sign such as fuzziness and cranky as the tooth is popping through. Therefore one baby varies to another that one could have peaceful sleep, while others might have numerous night wakings while teething in progress.

You might heard that some experts claims that teething will not interrupt baby's sleep, however each baby is not the same to others and will have different pain tolerances.

To understand as to how teething is affecting them and to have sympathetic to them, would be your job as parents. And not to forget also that you might want to make sure they get enough sleep.

There are two areas that are affected in your baby's sleep from his teething:

Early wakings in the morning. When teething, your baby might wake up earlier than usual and find it hard to be able to return himself to sleep.

Hard to nap. Teething baby takes longer to fall asleep at nap time and shorter nap. It is also possible that he might skip nap too. This can happen for a few days up to one week. Just remember that it is temporary so you don't have to stress.

These are a few notes that you need to know in handling your baby sleep problem when he is in teething phase:

As a baby's teething can take up to two years of age and it can be on and off, it would be better to have a plan on how you will handle the situation, which in this case the sleeping problem from your loved one. You need to consider not only your loved one condition where he is tired to have restless night as he is in pain, but also yourself and other family member that can have a disrupted night sleep too. The peak will last for about 2 to 4 days and at these times, your baby will need extra shooting until the tooth appear out of his gum.

You can give him Motrin, or if you are in Australia, people always use Bonjela and those two are proved to be quite effective. However, before giving any medication to your baby, please check first with your child's doctor about the dosage and other factor.

Expect your baby wants to feed more if you breastfeed him as it gives comfort mentally and also to their gums.

You can still continue your baby's sleep training during his teething phase. But perhaps be a little bit gentle and flexible to him in those 2-4 days peak time.

Getting baby to sleep through the is easier than you think!

Know your options will let you know what to do and hence avoid getting stressed or frustrated.

How Do Attachment Parenting and Baby Sleep Training Work Together?

Parents who practice or who want to practice attachment parenting often struggle with the concepts of how to sleep train their baby and how to help their baby sleep through the night. One of the primary principles of attachment parenting promotes the belief that sleep training techniques, primarily, crying it out, can have adverse psychological and physiological effects on the child. With attachment parenting, co-sleeping is strongly encouraged to ensure that baby's needs are being meet at night including helping to soothe them at night when they wake.

The common misconception is that sleep training only includes letting your baby cry it out as a way to learn to self soothe and put themselves to sleep. This is not true. There are other methods for getting your baby or toddler to sleep through the night and learning how to fall asleep on their own.

The elements of attachment parenting are designed to help baby and parent form strong and healthy attachments in part by tuning in to what babies need and responding appropriately. Helping your baby to learn how to sleep and have healthy sleep habits are part of tuning into what a baby needs. Helping your baby sleep through the night or helping your baby nap longer is being responsive to your baby's need for sleep. It is also important to keep in mind that not all babies are the same. The different temperaments of babies will play a role in how effective a sleep training method will work. For babies that have a more persistent or strong-willed temperament, a no-cry sleep solution can often be more effective.

Parents who practice attachment parenting are very passionate about this style of parenting. However, most people will agree that any type of parenting that promotes healthy and positive relationships is good for babies and families. Each family needs to find what works for them and for some families this involves sleep training their baby even as they practice attachment parenting. Sleep training can take into account a variety of parenting styles, including attachment parenting.

What is a mom to do when she is waking up many times a night with a breastfeeding, pacifier-demanding, or rocking-addicted baby? Sleep coaching can be essential to restoring a family balance.

Sleep training does NOT have to mean controlled crying or cry it out or any other variation of it. Attachment parenting parents potty train (baby led mostly), so why can't you sleep train? The obvious difference between potty training and sleep training is that potty training usually happens when the child is a toddler and sleep training may occur at a younger age. However, if you can potty train gently, you can sleep train gently, too. Once you understand the mechanics of sleep associations, then it is possible to create a sleep coaching plan that does not involve leaving baby to cry it out.

It can be unrealistic though to expect that there will not be any crying while your baby is learning how to fall asleep on his own, but you never have to leave your baby alone. Babies cry to communicate a need and sometimes they are crying because they are frustrated at not being able to sleep or because they are not getting enough sleep. Some crying can actually help lead babies to better sleeping. Often babies need to gain the confidence to believe that they can fall asleep without your assistance. This may mean that you have to give your child the room to learn to healthy sleep habits without the crutches of breastfeeding, pacifying or rocking to sleep. It is okay to remain close to encourage support during the transition during the times your baby is crying during sleep training. A baby who is not yet self soothing himself to sleep does not necessarily mean that he cannot self soothe if given the opportunity to learn and practice this skill.

When mom and baby are suffering from sleep deprivation, then sleep training is always worth a try and you can always re-evaluate if your plan does not go well. There is hope that you can possibly make a difference in your and your baby's life by "sleep coaching" even when you are "attachment parenting."

Choosing the Best Sleep Training Method

Want your baby to sleep through the night? Learn about five popular sleep training methods, and get some helpful advice from real-life parents.

Early parenthood is plagued by sleep deprivation and around-the-clock newborn care. This phase doesn't last forever though, and babies can usually snooze through the night by 6 months of age. The key is finding a sleep training method that works for your family and practicing it consistently. Keep reading to learn about five different ways to sleep train, with tips from other parents who've been through it too.

5 Popular Sleep Training Methods

The best sleep training method for your family depends on personal preference, so do your research before choosing one. Here are five of the most popular options.

Fading Method: With the fading sleep training method, parents rely on soothing techniques to help their baby fall asleep. These include feeding, rocking, snuggling, reading books, or singing lullabies. As your baby grows, they'll naturally become less needy, letting you slowly "fade out" of the nighttime routine. Fading is considered a gentle sleep training method.

This method works well for parents who cannot or do not want to see their baby cry. It involves little to no crying and works with your baby's natural sleep pattern. All you need to do is continue helping your baby fall asleep as usual. If you rock your baby, feed him or sing him for him to fall asleep, continue doing the same, but gradually reduce the timing, until you do it for less than a couple of minutes. This method calls for patience and time, but will teach your baby to fall asleep on his own.

This strategy involves temporarily moving your child's bedtime later while teaching him to fall asleep on his own. This can help use your child's natural sleep drive to make falling asleep easier. Usually I recommend moving the bedtime later by 30-60 minutes depending on prior experience. For example, if the family has previously tried to put their son down and he cried for 45 minutes before they gave up, I will move the bedtime 45 minutes later or more. There is evidence that removing the child from bed if they do not fall asleep after 15-20 minutes then putting them to bed again a few minutes later (a "response cost") is effective but I think that it is generally too complicated. Once your child can fall asleep within 15 minutes, you can move the bedtime earlier by 15 minutes every two days until you reach the desired bedtime (usually between 7:30-8:30 PM is best). It's important to avoid letting your child sleep in in the morning or falling asleep in the late afternoon in the stroller or the car, as they will be less tired at bedtime. This is one "gentle" sleep training method.

Avoiding "sneaky sleep" in the later afternoon.

Not allowing your child to sleep much later in the mornings, unless they are getting up at an uncomfortably early hour.

Cry It Out – Sleep Training Method for Babies

Experts believe that the ability to fall asleep on their own is an important life skill that babies must know and the 'crying it out method' is a good approach to sleep training which does just that. The idea behind the cry it out method is that by the time babies are six months or older, they are aware that crying results in being picked up, rocked and comforted, which leads to poor sleep associations during bedtime. But the CIO method discourages that and babies give up crying before bedtime within four or five nights of undergoing this training and learn to sleep on their own.

What is Cry It Out Method?

Cry it out method (CIO) is a sleep training approach devised for babies in which they are allowed to cry for a specific period of time before being comforted by the parent. CIO involves a variety of approaches and is often misunderstood as an approach where a baby is let alone to cry for as long as it takes before falling asleep. More appropriately called 'graduated extinction'; the idea behind it is to teach the baby to soothe herself to sleep when placed in bed without the presence of a parent.

Benefits of Cry It Out Method

As opposed to popular belief, practising CIO method does not mean that you are a 'bad parent' for letting your baby cry uncontrollably. In fact, the method is practised in a set pattern and has clear how-tos of going about it. CIO also has several benefits, some of which are listed below:

1. Lesser Stress on Babies

In a recent study conducted on infants trained in the CIO method, researchers found lower levels of cortisol, also known as the stress hormone. Decreased stress levels correlated with better sleep throughout the night with less or no disturbance in between.

2. Good for the Parent's Mental and Emotional Wellbeing

he same study tested for stress in parents, and found that not having to wake up at multiple times in the night to soothe their crying child, meant that the parents were lesser stressed as well. This improves their mental health and motivates them to be better at raising their infants.

3. Babies Fall Asleep Faster

CIO method starts showing results in a matter of days and after about a week of training, babies are known to fall asleep within 15 minutes of being in their crib. Experts believe that falling asleep alone is an important skill in life and the CIO makes it possible to develop that.

4. Does not Affect Baby's Long-term Behaviour or Social Skills

Contrary to popular belief, cry it out trained babies show no difference in behavioural traits and social skills from their non-cry counterparts as shown by long-term analysis.

5. Recommended by the American Academy of Paediatrics

The American Academy of Paediatrics considers CIO methods for infant sleep training as safe and recommends it to parents and physicians to try it out.

Theory Behind Cry It Out Method

The theory behind why cry it out works for babies is that when given the opportunity, it is possible for babies to fall asleep on their own and is a skill that can be mastered in time. A baby who is rocked or nursed to sleep every day won't learn to fall asleep on her own without these routines in place. This could be a problem when they wake up in the middle of the night as part of their regular sleep cycle. When they find that their parents are not around, it becomes a cause for concern and they stay awake and cry rather than going back to sleep.

On the other hand, babies trained in this method can soothe themselves to sleep when they wake up at night or during a nap. The method sees crying as a side effect and not the goal, as the baby gets used to sleeping on her own. At first, the training seems to make it worse, but the short-term discomfort endured by the baby and the parents is outweighed by the long-term benefits of a baby who sleeps effortlessly on her own and the parents getting a good night's rest.

Tips from Parents & Experts for Trying Cry It out Method

1. Discuss with your Partner and Develop a Plan

Both the parents need to be ready to cooperate and take turns to help each other out in the sleep training. It is best when both have enough time on their hands and are not caught up with work, business trips or visiting relatives that could upset the schedule. On the emotional front, both the partners need to have an understanding and how to proceed so they can support each other during rough patches.

2. Maintain a Bedtime Routine

With activities such as a bath, a lullaby or a book reading session, build activities up to the sleep time and maintain the routine so the child can get accustomed to it and fall asleep easily.

3. Prepare Yourself for Disappointments

Your baby may not be ready for the sleep training and it may not work initially. However, try again after a few weeks. There will be plenty of sleepless nights while the baby will wake up in the middle of the night and you will have to repeat the whole routine again.

4. Expect Relapses

Even when the baby is fully trained to sleep on a regular schedule, it might regress during times of illness or when travelling.

5. Stick to the Plan and Make It a Team Effort

Consistency is the key. Once the routine is established, it's important to follow through unless the baby isn't up to it physically or emotionally and then the training can be put on hold. Even when she wakes up in the middle of the night and the urge is strong to rock her to sleep, start over from square one. Discuss with your partner on taking turns and planning on what role each one of you plays during the training.

Do's and Don'ts of Cry It Out

Do explore other methods of sleep training and try the existing CIO methods with variations that suit you and your baby. Since all babies are different, and the same approach may not work for all, try a modification that works.

Do make sure that the child isn't crying for reasons such as hunger, pain or the need for a diaper change before bedtime.

Don't try the method with babies younger than six months of age. It is better to start with other gentler approaches while they are young.

Don't try CIO with babies that are sick or are teething. Babies tend to wake up in the middle of the night and the training would add to stress and anxiety.

Don't force the baby to adapt to the sleep routine. They may need some time to adapt to it and if it doesn't work the first time, give it a break and try again when they are a little older.

Drawbacks of Cry It Out

While there are pros and cons to this method, there isn't enough research done either way to support or to contradict the CIO approach strongly. Some of the drawbacks of the method are:

1. It May Cause Brain Damage

Ignoring your baby's cry might cause damage to the brain's neurons which can lead to hypersensitivity due to trauma in the long run. Since infants need to be frequently touched and given plenty of attention, the lack of it could alter the way in which the nervous system functions.

2. Babies Could have Prolonged Stress

Another body of research which challenges the 'low infant stress' hypothesis shows that babies undergoing CIO sleep training have elevated levels of the stress hormone cortisol. This persists even after sleeping and can have negative repercussions on the baby during her waking hours.

3. Affects Relationship between Parent and Baby

Crying is the mode through which babies communicate many of their needs and if it doesn't generate a positive response from the parents, the baby could develop a sense of detachment. The first two years are crucial for building a strong attachment with parents and detached infants could have insecurities growing up.

4. Could Affect Maternal Bonding

The CIO methods require mothers to override their maternal instincts to comfort their babies. This could lower her confidence in raising her child properly and erode the love and bonding between mother and child.

5. Could Increase the Risk of SIDS

The isolation of the CIO methods could increase the risk of Sudden Infant Death Syndrome (SIDS). Leaving an infant in a dark room with the door closed can lead to an unforeseen incident that can be fatal.

Can You Use CIO for Naps?

The Ferber method is primarily for night time sleep rather than naps during the day. As they get older, babies sleep less during the day. Therefore, the method is useful for a full night's sleep and babies trained in CIO can nap on their own.

Can Baby Sleep With Pacifiers & Toys?

The Ferber method recommends against the use of toys or pacifiers or any other object that babies may identify with sleep. Toys also pose a choking hazard while the baby is left alone and increase the risk of SIDS. However, the American Academy of Paediatrics recommends the use of pacifiers during bedtime and the choice is entirely yours depending on what works well for your baby.

The cry it out method may not be suitable for all parents and babies, but it has been effective for many. Although hearing your baby cry for a long time can be torturous, a little pain initially can yield plenty of good night's sleep for you and your baby.

How Long To Leave Your Baby

The key to the success of the cry it out method is consistency. Knowing the amount of time to wait in between checking on your baby is hugely important. The recommendations are to begin with a three minute wait, then five, then ten. On the second night, start with five then ten, then twelve. As each night progresses, make the initial interval longer and extend from there. However, these intervals, along with the Cry It Out method itself, are just guidelines. If you have any questions or worries in regard to baby sleep training, it's best to talk to your child's healthcare provider immediately. It's important to choose times your feel comfortable with, but also to stick to them and to extend them over time.

Benefits Of The Cry It Out Method

Potentially Causes Babies Less Stress. A recent study found that babies sleep trained with the cry it out method have less cortisol (a stress-linked hormone) than those trained with other methods.

Babies Fall Asleep Faster. After a week of the cry it out method, babies tend to be able to fall asleep in under fifteen minutes.

Good For Parents. The combination of knowing exactly when it's right to check on the baby combined with the overall higher amount of sleep means parents who are implementing the method are less stressed, anxious and sleep deprived.

Lack Of Proof Of Negative Social And Emotional Effects. In spite of what some may think, there is generally little evidence that cry it out trained babies have any differences in social skills or emotional state than other babies. But again, the research isn't conclusive.

Cry It Out Method Alternatives

The two main alternatives to the cry it out method are called the no tears method and the fading method. The no tears method is in direct opposition to the cry it out, while the fading method is somewhat of a hybrid of the two.

The no tears method was established in response to the cry it out method, by families for whom it hadn't worked. It relies on a fairly quick response by parents to any crying by their baby.

The fading method acts as a bridge between the two methods – the parents gradually diminishes or "fades" their role in helping their baby get to sleep. Advocates say it promotes independence of the baby while allowing a trusting and close relationship between parent and child.

Cry It Out Method Research

A study by the university of Adelaide showed that both the cry it out and the fading method had a positive impact on a child's ability to fall asleep. The same study showed sleep trained babies had lower levels of cortisol, the stress hormone. An earlier study at the same university found that after six years, here doesn't seem to be a huge amount of difference between sleep trained and non sleep trained kids supporting the hypothesis that the best sleep training method is the one which works for you.

Tips For Implementing The Cry It Out Method

Get Into A Routine. The best way to get your baby comfortable with any sleep training method is to get them into a good night time routine. Have a few steps that signal to your baby that it's nearly bedtime, like a bath, a bedtime story and a lullaby. This will help mentally prepare your baby for their coming bedtime, and thus they less likely to be taken by surprise and upset by it.

Prepare And Plan. Know that the first few nights of the cry it out method are likely to be tricky. You'll probably lose a little sleep, so for those who work weeks, it might be a good idea to begin the program on a Friday. Try as best you can to emotionally prepare yourself for the tricky first nights, too.

Stick With It. The main reason for failure of the cry it out method is parents giving up too quickly. While leaving your baby to cry can be irritating and even traumatic, undoing all your hard work by giving up will mean it's all for nothing.

Accept Some Early Difficulty. Not only will the cry it out method be difficult, sometimes you'll find it impossible. Forgive yourself for early relapses and try to get back into routine as quickly as possible.

Adapt The Method To Fit You. If the idea of three minutes of crying seems unfeasibly long, wait for fewer minutes before checking in. If you want to stretch the trajectory out and try to train over two weeks instead of just one, that's fine too. Make the method work for you, rather than the other way around.

What Is the Ferber Method of Sleep Training?

You've made the decision to sleep train your baby so you can (finally) start getting a little more shut-eye yourself. If you're looking into different plans and approaches, the Ferber method might be on your list of possible contenders.

The Ferber method of sleep training has been around for more than three decades, and it's helped countless little ones learn how to drift off to dreamland on their own. So should you give "Ferberizing" a try?

Here's how the Ferber method works and exactly how to do it, along with some smart tips that will help your baby get the hang of falling asleep solo sooner.

What is the Ferber Method?

The Ferber method is a form of cry it out sleep training (also known as "graduated extinction") developed by pediatric sleep expert Dr. Richard Ferber. It teaches babies to self-soothe, so they can fall asleep on their own and fall back to sleep when they wake up during the night.

Some parents who sleep train with cry it out opt not to go back into their baby's room at all, even if the baby cries for a long time. The Ferber method is considered to be a gentler option, since it involves periodically checking in on your baby when she's crying.

During the check-ins, you'll go to your baby at timed intervals that gradually get longer until she falls asleep. The check-ins also get longer on subsequent nights. Ferber calls it the "progressive waiting approach."

You can soothe your baby verbally or give her a gentle rub or pat. But you shouldn't pick her up or feed her, and your visits should only last a minute or two.

How do you do the Ferber Method?

Even though sleep training can sometimes feel hard emotionally, the actual steps of the Ferber method are simple and straightforward. Here's what you'll do:

After your bedtime routine, put your baby into her crib. She should be drowsy but awake.

Tell your baby goodnight and leave the room.

If your baby cries, wait for a set amount of time (more on how long below), then go back in to briefly comfort her by talking in a soothing voice or gently patting her. Don't pick her up or feed her.

Leave the room and repeat as needed if your baby continues to cry, going back in to reassure her at specific timed intervals.

When should you start the Ferber method on your baby?

Babies are generally ready for sleep training, including methods like Ferber, around 5 or 6 months. At that point, they're developmentally capable of self-soothing. They're also old enough to sleep through the night without eating.

But if you have questions or aren't sure whether your little one is quite there yet, don't hesitate to bring it up with her pediatrician.

You don't have to sleep train as soon as your baby hits the 5- or 6-month mark. If you'd feel more comfortable holding off until your little one is a bit older, that's okay. Just keep in mind that the older your baby gets, the harder it might be for her to learn to fall asleep on her own instead of being rocked, fed or soothed by you.

Ferber Method Chart

The Ferber method is considered a gentler form of cry it out sleep training, since it lets you check in on your baby at timed intervals to comfort her (with soft words and touches) when she's crying.

In his book Solve Your Child's Sleep Problems (which parents trying this method might want to borrow or buy), Ferber recommends doing check-ins at the following times:

Day 1

First check-in after: 3 minutes

Second check-in after: 5 minutes

Third check-in after: 10 minutes

Subsequent check-in after: 10 minutes

Day 2

First check-in after: 5 minutes

Second check-in after: 10 minutes

Third check-in after: 12 minutes

Subsequent check-in after: 12 minutes

Day 3

First check-in after: 10 minutes

Second check-in after: 12 minutes

Third check-in after: 15 minutes

Subsequent check-in after: 15 minutes

Day 4

First check-in after: 12 minutes

Second check-in after: 15 minutes

Third check-in after: 17 minutes

Subsequent check-in after: 17 minutes

Day 5

First check-in after: 15 minutes

Second check-in after: 17 minutes

Third check-in after: 20 minutes

Subsequent check-in after: 20 minutes

Day 6

First check-in after: 17 minutes

Second check-in after: 20 minutes

Third check-in after: 25 minutes

Subsequent check-in after: 25 minutes

Day 7

First check-in after: 20 minutes

Second check-in after: 25 minutes

Third check-in after: 30 minutes

Subsequent check-in after: 30 minutes

Here's a Ferber method chart that's easy to check and refer to:

How long does the Ferber sleep method take to work on your baby?

All babies respond to sleep training in their own way, and some take to the new bedtime routine a little faster than others. But in general, you can expect the crying to diminish steadily over three nights or so. And sometime between nights four and seven, it will likely stop altogether.

Does that mean your baby will never cry at bedtime or wake up in the middle of the night again? Even after sleep training, it's normal for your little one to hit the occasional rough patch like when she's sick, teething or even working on a big developmental milestone.

But now that sleep training has given her a solid foundation, it should be relatively easy for her to get back to her usual snooze routine once the issue has passed.

Ferber sleep Method Training Tips

The sleep training process isn't exactly fun, but it doesn't have to be a nightmare either.

To set the stage for success and maybe have everyone sleeping blissfully through the night a little sooner keep these strategies in mind.

Be smart about your start time. Sleep training can be a big deal for both you and your baby, so block out time on the calendar when everything else is relatively calm. If your little one is sick or teething, or if you've got a new babysitter starting or you're going back to work, it's worth holding off until things have settled back down. Avoid sleep training on vacation too travel will only derail your efforts.

Wean nighttime feedings. It can be harder for your baby to get the hang of sleep training if you sometimes respond to her cries by going in to feed her.

Establish a bedtime routine, if you haven't already. Soothing activities like a bath, book and snuggles will help your baby wind down for the night. If your bedtime routine currently ends with a feeding, try moving it earlier so there's no risk of your baby falling asleep at the breast or bottle. Remember, she should be drowsy but awake when you put her in the crib.

Watch for your baby's sleepy cues. You want to get your baby into bed when she's nice and tired but not overtired. Your little one will have a harder time settling down once she's past the point of exhaustion. And she might be more likely to sleep restlessly and wake throughout the night.

Stick with the crib for bedtime and naps. At night, the crib is the most obvious place for sleep. But if your baby is in the habit of napping in places other than her crib, she might have a harder time sleeping well in it at night too.

Make sure both parents are on board and consider having your partner handle check-ins. It's important that both you and your partner agree to try the Ferber method of sleep training, as you'll need each other for support during the process. And if your baby associates you with feeding and comfort, having Dad or a partner go in might help her settle down a little easier.

Be consistent. Listening to your baby cry can be hard, and it might even tempt you to abandon your plan. But sticking with it will help her get the hang of things faster — so you all can rest easier.

When to stop trying the Ferber Method

Cry it out methods like the Ferber method can be a great tool for helping babies become great sleepers. But if after a week or two, your baby hasn't made much progress or it seems like she's still crying a lot, it might be time to take a break.

You could try the Ferber method again a little later on, or switch gears and try another sleep training approach. It's also worth talking with your baby's pediatrician. She can help rule out any underlying issues that might be making it harder for your baby to sleep, like infant acid reflux, teething or an ear infection.

The Ferber method of sleep training can help your baby learn how to fall asleep on her own and soothe herself back to sleep when she wakes during the night. As with most sleep training approaches, there will probably be some tears.

But if you're consistent, the crying will decrease after just a few days. And within a week or two she and you will be getting a better night's sleep.

The Chair Sleep Training Method

The Chair Method involves more tears than the previous two; however, you don't leave your baby unattended in the room at all.

First, start by doing your bedtime routine and turn on the white noise. Then, put a chair very near the crib, bassinet, or bed. You will sit on the chair as your baby falls asleep.

The goal is not to help your child fall asleep, nor to help her calm down necessarily, depending on how you implement it. You are generally not supposed to give your child any attention. The reason you are in the chair is only to reassure them that you are there and have not left them alone. Each night you gradually move the chair further away from them until you are right outside the door until eventually, you no longer need the chair at all.

As you might suspect, this method can be very difficult, depending on temperament, and can take many days or weeks. It can be difficult to avoid engaging with your child and "watching them cry" is very difficult. Furthermore, it can be a little confusing to the child (particularly younger ones) when you don't interact. However, with time and consistency, this can be a good option for parents who do not want to leave their child alone to cry but who haven't had success with other methods, either.

There are variations to this method (such as Kim West's Sleep Lady Shuffle) where you do tend to the baby periodically, verbally and/or physically, and then go back to your chair. As with many things, finding what works best for you and your child is key.

Q: What age for The Chair Method?

Our recommendation is over 3-6 months old, depending on how severe the sleep disruptions have been. Since it's a gentler method, you can try it with just about any age baby or toddler. Of course, if your toddler is already in a bed of which he can get out, this might not be the easiest to use.

The Pick-Up-Put-Down Sleep Training Method (PUPD)

The Pick-Up-Put-Down Method is another gentle sleep training method. The PUPD method works just the way it sounds: when it's time to sleep, and your baby is fussing or crying in his crib or bassinet, you pick him up and comfort him until he's calm and drowsy. Then, you put him back in his crib to sleep, repeating this cycle until your baby is finally asleep. Pick-Up-Put-Down is another method that requires quite a bit of patience, depending on your baby, and it won't work for every baby; some babies find being picked up and put down so often over-stimulating, and they gradually become frustrated and worked up, instead of relaxed

This is a no-cry sleep training method. Simply pick up your baby whenever they cry, and put them back down after soothing. Repeat these steps until the little one falls asleep. This is a no-cry sleep training method. Simply pick up your baby whenever they cry, and put them back down after soothing. Repeat these steps until the little one falls asleep.

This method is pretty straightforward. The idea is to pick the baby up from the crib when he is fussy and cries during bedtime. Comfort him until he's calm and ready to get back into the crib. You will need to repeat this method until the baby falls asleep. This is a gentle method that will assure the baby that you are around. However, it can require a good amount of patience and may not be ideal for all babies. Some babies may even feel worked up due to the constant picking up.

Develop a realistic attitude about Nighttime Parenting

Sleeping, like eating, is not a state you can force a baby into. The best you can do is to create a secure environment that allows sleep to overtake your baby. A realistic long- term goal is to help your baby develop a healthy attitude about sleep. Baby should feel that sleep is a pleasant state to enter and a secure state to remain in. Many sleep problems in older children and adults stem from children growing up with an unhealthy attitude about sleep. Such as sleep was not a pleasant state to enter and was a fearful state to remain in. Just as daytime parenting is a long-term investment, so is nighttime parenting. Teach your baby a restful attitude about sleep when they are young. By doing this, both you and your children will sleep better when they are older.

Beware of Sleep Trainers

Ever since parenting books found their way into the nursery, sleep trainers have touted magic formulas promising to get babies to sleep through the night – for a price and at a risk. Most of these sleep-training techniques are just variations of the old cry-it-out method. And technology has found its way into nighttime baby care by providing tired parents with a variety of sleep-inducing gadgets. These gadgets are designed to lull a baby off to sleep alone in her crib: oscillating cradles, crib vibrators that mimic a car ride, and teddy bears that "breathe." All promise to fill in for parents on night duty. Be discerning about using someone else's method to get your baby to sleep. Before trying any sleep-inducing program, you be the judge.

Run these schemes through your inner sensitivity before trying them on your baby, especially if they involve leaving your baby alone to cry:

Does this advice sound sensible, will it fit your baby's temperament and does it feel right to you?

If your current daytime or nighttime routine is not working for you, think about what changes you can make in yourself and your lifestyle that will make it easier for you to meet your baby's needs. This is a better approach than immediately trying to change your baby. After all, you can control your own reactions to a situation. You can't control how your baby reacts. Use discernment about advice that promises a sleep-through-the-night more convenient baby. These programs involve the risk of creating a distance between you and your baby and undermining the mutual trust between parent and child.

Stay flexible when putting baby to Sleep

No single approach will work with all babies all the time or even all the time with the same baby. Don't persist with a failing experiment. If the "sleep program" isn't working for your family, drop it. Develop a nighttime parenting style that works for you. Babies have different nighttime temperaments and families have varied lifestyles.

Keep working at a style of nighttime parenting that fits the temperament of your baby and your own lifestyle. If it's working, stick with it. If it's not, be open to trying other nighttime parenting styles. And, be prepared for one style of nighttime parenting to work at one stage of an infant's life, yet need a change as she enters another stage. Be open to trying different nighttime approaches. Follow your heart rather than some stranger's sleep-training advice, and you and your baby will eventually work out the right nighttime parenting style for your family.

Decide where baby sleeps Best

There is no right or wrong place for babies to sleep. Wherever all family members sleep the best is the right arrangement for you and your baby. Some babies sleep best in their own crib in their own room, some sleep better in their own bassinet or crib in the parents' bedroom, other babies sleep best snuggled right next to mommy in the parents' bed. Many parents prefer a co-sleeper arrangement. Realistically, most parents use various sleeping arrangements at various stages during the infant's first two years. Be open to changing styles as baby's developmental needs and your family situation changes.

Conditioning Baby to Fall Asleep

Sleep is not a state you can force your baby into. Sleep must naturally overtake your baby. Your nighttime parenting role is to set the conditions that make sleep attractive and to present cues that suggest to baby that sleep is expected. Try the following sleep tight tips, which may vary at different stages in your baby's development. What doesn't work one week may work the next.

Get baby used to a variety of Sleep Associations

The way an infant goes to sleep at night is the way she expects to go back to sleep when she awakens. So, if your infant is always rocked or nursed to sleep, she will expect to be rocked or nursed back to sleep. Sometimes nurse her off to sleep, sometimes rock her off to sleep, sometimes sing her off to sleep, and sometimes use tape recordings, and switch off with your spouse on putting her to bed. There are two schools of thought on the best way to put babies to sleep: the parent-soothing method and the self-soothing method. Both have advantages and possible disadvantages:

1. Parent-soothing method. When baby is ready to sleep, a parent or other caregiver helps baby make a comfortable transition from being awake to falling asleep, usually by nursing, rocking, singing, or whatever comforting techniques work.

Advantages:

Baby learns a healthy sleep attitude – that sleep is a pleasant state to enter and a secure state to remain in.

Creates fond memories about being parented to sleep.

Builds parent-infant trust

Disadvantages:

Because of the concept of sleep associations, baby learns to rely on an outside prop to get to sleep, so as the theory goes when baby awakens he will expect help to get back to sleep. This may exhaust the parents.

2. Self-soothing method: Baby is put down awake and goes to sleep by himself. Parents

If baby learns to go to sleep by himself, he may be better able to put himself back to sleep without parental help, because he doesn't associate going to sleep with parents comforting. May be tough on baby, but eventually less exhausting for parents.

Disadvantages:

Involves a few nights of let-baby-cry-it-out

Risks baby losing trust

Seldom works for high-need babies with persistent personalities

Overlooks medical reasons for night waking

Remember: In working out your own parenting-to-sleep techniques and rituals, be sensitive to the nighttime needs of your individual baby and remember your ultimate goal: to create a healthy sleep attitude in your baby and to get all family members a restful night's sleep.

Daytime Mellowing

A peaceful daytime is likely to lead to a restful night. The more attached you are to your baby during the day and the more baby is held and calmed during the day, the more likely this peacefulness is to carry through into the night. If your baby has a restless night, take inventory of unsettling circumstances that may occur during the day: Are you too busy? Are the daycare and the daycare provider the right match for your baby? Does your baby spend a lot of time being held and in-arms by a nurturant caregiver, or is he more of a "crib baby" during the day? We have noticed babies who are carried in baby slings for several hours a day settle better at night. Babywearing mellows the infant during the day, behavior that carries over into restfulness at night.

Set Predictable and Consistent nap Routines

Pick out the times of the day that you are most tired, for example, 11:00 a.m. and 4:00 p.m. Lie down with your baby at these times every day for about a week to get your baby used to a daytime nap routine. This also sets you up to get some much-needed daytime rest rather than be tempted to "finally get something done" while baby is napping. Babies who have consistent nap routines during the day are more likely to sleep longer stretches at night.

Consistent Bedtimes and Rituals

Babies who enjoy consistent bedtimes and familiar going-to-sleep rituals usually go to sleep easier and stay asleep longer. Yet, because of modern lifestyles, consistent and early bedtimes are not as common, or realistic, as they used to be. Busy two-income parents often don't get home until six or seven o'clock in the evening, so it's common for older babies and toddlers to procrastinate the bedtime ritual. This is prime time with their parents and they are going to milk it for all they can get.

In some families, a later afternoon nap and a later bedtime is more practical. Familiar bedtime rituals set the baby up for sleep. The sequence of a warm bath, rocking, nursing, lullabies, etc. set the baby up to feel that sleep is expected to follow. Capitalize on a principle of early infant development: patterns of association. Baby's developing brain is like a computer, storing thousands of sequences that become patterns. When baby clicks into the early part of the bedtime ritual, he is programmed for the whole pattern that results in drifting off to sleep.

Calming Down

Give baby a warm bath followed by a soothing massage to relax tense muscles and busy minds. Be careful, though, because this will stimulate some babies.

Tank up your baby during the day

Babies need to learn that daytime is for eating and nighttime is mostly for sleeping. Some older babies and toddlers are so busy playing during the day that they forget to eat and make up for it during the night by waking frequently to feed. To reverse this habit, feed your baby at least every three hours during the day to cluster the baby's feedings during the waking hours. Upon baby's first night waking, attempt a full feeding, otherwise some babies, especially breastfed infants, get in the habit of nibbling all night.

Transitioning Techniques

Many infants need help making the transition from being awake to falling asleep, which is really a prolongation of the bedtime ritual that conditions baby that sleep is expected to soon follow.

Nursing Down

Nestle next to your baby and breastfeed or bottle-feed him off to sleep. The smooth continuum from a warm bath, to warm arms, to warm breast, to warm bed is a recipe for sleep to soon follow.

Fathering Down

Place baby in the neck nestle position (nestle baby's head against the front of your neck with your chin against the top of baby's head. The vibration of the deeper male voice lulls baby to sleep) and rock your baby to sleep. If baby doesn't drift off to sleep while rocking, lie down with your baby, still in the neck nestle position, and let baby temporarily fall asleep draped over your chest. Once baby is asleep, ease the sleeping baby into his bed and sneak away.

Rocking or Walking Down

Try rocking baby to sleep in a bedside rocking chair, or walk with baby, patting her back and singing or praying.

Nestling Down

For some babies, the standard fall-to-sleep techniques are not enough. Baby just doesn't want to be put down to sleep alone. After rocking or feeding baby to sleep in your arms, lie down with your sleeping baby next to you and nestle close to her until she is sound asleep. We call this the "teddy- bear snuggle."

Wearing Down

Some babies are so revved up during the day that they have trouble winding down at night. Place your baby in a baby sling and wear her around the house for a half-hour or so before the designated bedtime. When she is fully asleep (see limp-limb sign) in the sling, ease her out of the sling onto her bed. For babies who are used to nursing off to sleep in a mother's arms, fathers can wear their baby down to sleep and give mother a break. Wearing down is particularly useful for the reluctant napper. When baby falls asleep in the sling, snuggled with his tummy against your chest, or draped over your chest once you lie down, you both can take a much-needed nap.

Swinging down

Wind-up swings for winding down babies are a boon to parents who have neither the time, energy, or creativity to muster up rituals of their own. Tired parents will pay anything for a good night's sleep. Once in awhile a moving plastic seat may be more sleep-inducing than a familiar pair of arms. Sometimes high-need babies associate a parent's body with play and stimulation and will not drift off to sleep in a human swing. For them, the mechanical one is less stimulating, if not downright boring, and therefore can be a useful part of a sleep-ritual repertoire.

Yet remember, high-need babies are notoriously resistant to mechanical mother substitutes and will usually protest anything less than the real mom. Before you actually spend money on a swing, you might want to borrow one for a week or two to see if the spell of the swing will last. You may discover that you are uncomfortable with mechanical mothering and decide to get more creative. Still, swings have their moments.

Driving down

If you've tried all the above transitioning techniques and baby still resists falling asleep, place baby in a carseat and drive around until she falls asleep. When you return home and baby is in a deep sleep, carry the carseat (with the sleeping baby) into your bedroom and let baby remain in the carseat until the first nightwaking. If she is in a deep sleep (witness the limp-limb sign hands unclenched, arms dangling loosely at her side, facial muscles still), you may be able to ease her out of the carseat into her own bed.

Mechanical Mothers

Gadgets to put and keep baby asleep are becoming big business. Tired parents pay high prices for a good night's sleep. It's all right to use these as relief when the main comforter wears out, but a steady diet of these artificial sleep inducers may be unhealthy. We remember a newspaper article extolling the sleep-tight virtues of a teddy bear, with a tape player in his stuffing that sings or makes breathing sounds. Baby can snuggle up to the singing, breathing, synthetic bear. Personally, we are not keen on our babies going to sleep to someone else's canned voice. Why not use the real parent?

Stay Asleep Techniques

Now that you've learned all the tricks of the nighttime trade to get your baby to sleep, here are some ways to keep your baby asleep. Because of the characteristics of babies' sleep cycles and easy arousability from sleep, you will notice that we purposely omit what we call the "harden your heart" method: put your baby down to sleep awake in a crib in his own room, put cotton in your ears, and let him cry himself to sleep. When he awakens, don't go into him. He will soon learn to put himself to sleep and back to sleep. We believe that this method is unsafe, runs the risk of baby losing trust, and, for infants with persistent personalities, doesn't work. Try these tips to help your baby sleep increasingly longer stretches at night.

Dress for the Occasion

Try various ways of swaddling your baby at night. In the early months, many babies like to "sleep tight," securely swaddled in a cotton baby blanket. Older infants like to sleep "loose," and may sleep longer stretches with loose coverings that allow them more freedom of movement. Oftentimes, dressing a baby loosely during the day, but swaddling him at night, conditions the baby to associate sleep with swaddling. A baby who gets too hot or too cold may become restless. Adjust the layering according to the temperature of the room and the sleep habits of your baby. Allergy-prone babies sleep better in 100 percent cotton sleepwear.

Quiet in the Bedroom

Since most babies can block out disturbing noise, you don't have to create a noiseless sleeping environment, yet some babies startle and awaken easily with sudden noises. For these babies, oil the joints and springs of a squeaky crib, put out the dog before he barks and turn the ringer off on the phone.

Darkness in the Bedroom

Use opaque shades to block out the light, which may get you an extra hour of sleep if you have one of those little roosters who awakens to the first ray of sunlight entering the bedroom.

Sounds to Sleep by

Repetitive, nearly monotonous sounds that lull baby to sleep are known as white noise, such as the sounds of a fan, air conditioner, or even tape recordings of womb sounds or vacuum cleaner sounds. Also, try running water from a nearby faucet or shower, a bubbling fish tank, a loudly ticking clock, or a metronome set at sixty beats a minute. (These can all be tape-recorded.) Try music to sleep by, such as tape recordings of waterfalls or ocean sounds, or a medley of easy-listening lullabies on a continuous-play tape recorder. These sleep-inducing sounds remind baby of the sounds she was used to hearing in the womb.

Music to Sleep by

Try a continuous-play tape recording of your baby's favorite lullabies, so when she awakens she can resettle herself to the familiar sleep-inducing sound of the tape-recording. You can make a medley of your own lullabies that have been proven sleep-inducers.

Leave a little bit of mother behind

If you have a separation-sensitive baby, leave a breast pad in the cradle, or play a continuous tape recording of yourself singing a bedtime lullaby.

A full Tummy (but not too full)

While stuffing baby with a glob of cereal before bedtime seldom works, it may be worth a try. A tablespoon or two given to a baby over six months of age may get you an extra hour or two. Tiny babies have tiny tummies, a bit bigger than the size of their fist. So, your baby's digestive system was designed for small, frequent feedings, which is why, in the early months, babies feed at least every 3 to 4 hours at night and more often during the day. (See Foods for Sleep)

Clear the Nose

In the early months, babies need clear nasal passages to breathe. Later they can alternatively breathe through their mouth if their nose is blocked. Bedroom inhalant allergies are a common cause of stuffy noses and consequent night waking. Dust-free your baby's bedroom as much as possible. (Remove fuzzy blankets, down comforters, dust-collecting fuzzy toys, etc.) If your baby is particularly allergy-prone, a HEPA-type air filter will help. As an added nighttime perk, the "white noise" from the hum of the air filter may help baby stay asleep.

Relieve Teething Pain

Even though you may not yet be able to feel baby's teeth, teething discomfort may start as early as three months and continue off and on all the way through the two-year molars. A wet bed sheet under baby's head, a drool rash on the cheeks and chin, swollen and tender gums, and a slight fever are telltale clues that teething is the nighttime culprit. What to do? With your doctor's permission, give appropriate doses of acetaminophen just before parenting your baby to sleep and again in four hours if baby awakens.

Change wet or Soiled Diapers

Some babies are bothered by wet diapers at night, most are not. If your baby sleeps through wet diapers, there is no need to awaken her for a change. However, if you're treating a persistent diaper rash, continue to change them. Nighttime bowel movements necessitate a change. If possible, change the diapers just before feeding, as baby is likely to fall asleep during or after feeding. Some breastfed babies, however, have a bowel movement during or immediately after feeding. In that case, baby will need changing again. If you are using cloth diapers, putting two or three diapers on your baby before bedtime will decrease the sensation of wetness.

Remove Irritating Sleepwear

Some babies cannot settle in synthetic sleepwear. A mother in our practice went through our whole checklist of night waking causes until she discovered her baby was sensitive to polyester sleepers. Once she changed to 100 percent cotton clothing, her baby slept better. Besides being restless, some babies show skin allergies. A rash may appear due to new clothing, detergents, and fabric softeners.

Remove Airborne Irritants

Environmental irritants may cause congested breathing passages and awaken baby. Common household examples are cigarette smoke, baby powder, paint fumes, hair spray, animal dander (keep animals out of an allergic child's bedroom), plants, clothing (especially wool), stuffed animals, dust from a bed canopy, feather pillows, blankets, and fuzzy toys that collect lint and dust. If your baby consistently awakens with a stuffy nose, suspect irritants or allergens in the bedroom.

A warm Bed

Placing a warm baby onto cold sheets can cause trouble. Especially in cold weather, use flannel sheets or place a warm towel on the sheets to warm them. But be sure to remove the towel before placing baby on the warmed sheets.

Create the right Bedroom Temperature and Humidity

A consistent bedroom temperature of around 70 degrees F is preferable. Also, relative humidity of around 50 percent is most conducive to sleep. Dry air may leave baby with a stuffy nose that awakens him. Yet, too high a humidity fosters allergy-producing molds. A warm-mist vaporizer in your baby's sleeping area helps maintain an adequate and consistent relative humidity. This can especially help during the winter months. (And, the "white noise" of a consistent hum may help baby stay asleep.)

What to do when baby Wakes

When your baby awakens, develop a nighttime parenting approach. An Approach that respects your baby's need for nighttime trust and comfort, in addition to the need for baby and parents to quickly get back to sleep. While some babies are self-soothers, being able to resettle easily and quickly without outside help, others (especially those high-need babies with more persistent personalities) need a helping hand (or breast, or whatever tool you can muster up at 3:00 a.m.). Try these back-to-sleep comforters:

Laying on of Hands

Determine what your baby's nighttime temperament is. Is your baby a born self-soother who awakens, whimpers, squirms, and then resettles by herself? Or is your baby, if not promptly attended to, one whose cries escalate and becomes angry and difficult to resettle? If you can get to your baby quickly before she completely awakens, you may be able to resettle her back to sleep with a firm laying on of hands. To add the finishing touch, pat your baby's back or bottom rhythmically to match your heartbeat. Remove your hands gradually first one and then the other – easing the pressure slowly so as not to startle baby awake. Sometimes fathers, perhaps because they have larger hands, are more successful in this hands-on ritual.

Honor your Partner with his share of Nighttime Parenting

It's important for babies to get used to father's way of comforting and being put to sleep (and back to sleep) in father's arms, otherwise, mothers burn out. A father's participation in nighttime parenting is especially important for the breastfeeding infant who assumes the luxury that "mom's diner" is open all night.

Detect hidden Medical causes of Night Waking

If you've tried all these techniques and your infant is still waking up frequently – and painfully – suspect there may be an underlying medical problem contributing to your baby's night waking. (See Hidden Causes of Night Waking) One of the most common hidden medical causes of night waking (and colicky behavior) in babies is a condition known as gastroesophageal reflux (GER). Due to a weakness of a circular band of muscle where the esophagus joins the stomach, irritating stomach acids are regurgitated into baby's esophagus. This causing pain like adults would call heartburn.

GER Clues

Clues that your baby may be suffering from GER are painful bursts of night waking fussiness, particularly after eating; frequent spitting up (although not all babies with GER spit up regularly); bouts of colicky, abdominal pain; frequent bouts of unexplained wheezing; and hearing throaty sounds after feeding. Another hidden medical cause of night waking is allergies to formula or dairy products. Such as milk-based formulas or in dairy products in a breastfeeding mother's diet. Clues that milk allergies may be causing night waking (and colicky behavior) are bloating, diarrhea, and a red rash around baby's anus, in addition to many of the signs described above under GER.

If your baby is not only waking up frequently but waking up "in pain," discuss these two medical possibilities with your doctor, since both can be diagnosed and treated, giving everyone in the family a more peaceful night's sleep. The above tools not only help your short-term goal of getting your baby to sleep but, more importantly, create a healthy sleep attitude that lasts a lifetime. A baby who enjoys this style of nighttime parenting learns that sleep is a pleasant state to enter and a secure state to remain in. Therein lies the key to nighttime parenting.

Should Babies Sleep With Their Parents?

Should you let babies and small children sleep in the bed with their parents and if so, for how long?

I raised four children and they all slept with us in a standard double bed up to a point--it was just easier that way. I'm a basically lazy person once I get bedded down for the night. I really hated getting up to feed and change junior. I'd lay out couple of clean diapers by the bed and a plastic bag for the dirties. The night-time snacks, of course, didn't require any special preparation--they were on tap. The babies slept on my side on the edge rather than the middle of the bed because my husband was afraid he would roll on them. I always threw down extra pillows on the floor on my side in case they either rolled or got pushed out.

But that is ME. A lot of factors enter into this decision: How sound you sleep, whether you are overweight, what medications you take, the size of your bed your child's temperament, your feelings and your spouse's feelings on the issue, what to do with baby when you are feeling amorous, is the crib in the parents' room or not, the absence or presence of siblings, and so on. A very heavy sleeper who takes meds (especially sleep meds) and/or is overweight might want to think twice about having the baby in the bed with them. There is no right and wrong here, and what is right in one situation may be wrong in another; what is right for one child may be wrong for another, Some people have very strong opinions on both sides of this issue. Some will try to make you feel like you are a horrible parent if you do it and some will try to make you feel horrible if you don't. Don't let them do it. You are the expert here. You can trust yourself that YOU are the best person to know.

We started encouraging ours to sleep in the crib when they started getting rowdy--the exact age was different from child to child, but generally around the age they could walk easily. We also expected them to be able to fall asleep on their own and trained them to do so by means of a trick I learned from a daycare provider: most babies fall asleep easily when their bottoms are rhythmically and surprisingly firmly (!) patted for about fifteen minutes, in or out of the parental bed. Once there were multiple children and they were beyond the age of needing sustenance every four hours they were quite happy to curl up with each other to sleep: big sis would crawl in the crib with little brother and once little brother learned to escape from the crib he would just as often crawl in with big sis, especially on a cold night.

I honestly think that whether children sleep with their parents or not is a non-issue. Here is my advice:

- ➤ Have confidence in your instincts
- ➤ Don't waver between the advice given in this book or that book
- ➤ Don't beat yourself up if feel you made a mistake -- children are forgiving
- ➤ Present a consistent and firm but loving presence to your little one (note: love is not the same thing as indulgence)

> ➤ Don't try to make him happy all the time, rather teach him how to make himself happy.

Is It Healthy To Let Your Baby Cry?

Babies Cry to Communicate Their Needs

The first thing to understand is that babies are not toddlers. Babies cry as a form of basic instinctive communication, not because they're trying to manipulate. Baby's brains are still developing and have not yet reached the ability to reason. They cry because they NEED something. Once you understand that they need something, the questions are: do you spoil them if you give them what they need? Should you fulfill those needs immediately? And will you create attachment issues if you meet their need for comfort and attention?

Do you spoil your baby if you give him what he needs?

First you have to ask yourself, what does "spoiling a child" mean? You spoil a child when you give that child what he wants and needs without having him work for those things himself. Obviously this only applies when the child is CAPABLE of acquiring his wants and needs for himself. Babies are not capable of giving themselves food, a diaper change, love, comfort, etc. They depend on you completely for these things. Since your baby is not capable of fulfilling his own needs, you are not spoiling him by doing it for him.

Should you fulfill those needs Immediately?

If you jump the instant your baby starts crying, will he learn to manipulate you? If you let him cry a little while before attending to his needs, will you teach him patience? The experts all agree that a baby's brain is not developed enough to understand the art of manipulation or grasp the concept of patience. You could try to teach your baby patience anyway. After all, some babies learn more quickly than others. What could it hurt? Consider what the reseachers said,

"Your ability to read and respond to your baby's emotions will lay a foundation of security and trust, helping him form relationships with other people and feel understood and accepted." It's possible you might be teaching your baby patience, but you may be doing it at the risk of him not feeling secure, not feeling trust for you and others, and not feeling understood and accepted.

Will you create attachment issues if you meet your baby's need for comfort and attention?

It's normal for your baby to be attached to you. After all, you carried him in your womb for 9 months. You are all that baby has known. However, there comes a point in time when it's not healthy or realistic for you to be with your baby, comforting and entertaining him 24/7. So should you give your baby comfort and attention every time he cries for it? I say absolutely! Remember that your baby is crying to communicate something to you. If he's saying he NEEDS comfort and attention, it's healthy to give it to him. It becomes unhealthy when you're giving your baby attention all the time, even when he doesn't ask for it. Give your baby alone time so he can see that he doesn't need you every second, but when he starts crying, know your baby is ready for some comfort and attention.

Sleep-Training

One of the reasons your baby cries is because he's tired and needs to sleep. Some experts will tell you that you can train your baby to fall asleep on his own if you let him cry when he's tired. They say that if you always rock your baby to sleep or do other things to help facilitate sleep, your baby will become dependent on this action for sleep in the future. However, Darcia Narvaez (Ph.D.), states in the book Let Crying Babes Lie? So Wrong that "letting babies cry who have specific needs creates harder to manage sleep routines and leaves infants with an overactive stress response system that would make settling of any sort even more difficult." Quite the opposite of what you're trying to accomplish! It's important to point out that even the experts who are for sleep-training caution against doing it before your child is 4 months old.

 After looking over all the information, it's my opinion that we should NOT let our babies cry without trying to fulfill their needs immediately. Babies can't manipulate, they can't reason, they can't learn patience. All they can do is tell us what they need by crying. Obviously the rules change when babies become older and develop new skills and understanding, but in the meantime, giving our babies what they need helps them to feel loved, safe, understood and accepted.

CHAPTER FOUR

Crying-It-Out Harms Babies Brains

"Crying-it-out Harms Babies Brains."

This media coverage is tough on the sleep deprived mother who hears that on the one hand that, if she doesn't do something about her sleepless baby, he will probably grow into a sleepless child who will have problems with his weight and/or behaviour. And on the other hand, if she allows him to cry until he figures out how to fall asleep by himself, it may harm his brain.

I think it's safe to say there's a middle ground, which might be called "common sense parenting". As parents we are faced with choices that we have to make on behalf of our children on a daily basis and these choices have to take into account the needs of our whole family.

In her new book, Leach argues, "It is potentially damaging to leave babies to cry..." because the crying generates high levels of the hormone cortisol, which, "neurobiologists say is toxic to the human brain". I am sure that allowing a six week old baby to cry for hours alone, day after day, could cause damage to his developing brain. I think it would be cruel to do that to an adult.

But our babies grow older and Leach says herself, "don't, for heaven's sake, leap to respond to a demanding one-year-old as you would to a newborn." In fact, what Leach warns against in her book is parents not responding to a baby who is crying, rather than not allowing a baby to cry. All babies cry, some more than others. What is important is that we respond appropriately.

I'm not a parenting guru, but I am a mother. I have suffered sleep deprivation for a few nights here and there. It's caused me to snap at the people I love and unreasonably lose my temper with my pre-schooler. I know how it feels to lose perspective, to become over emotional and irritable after a week of no sleep. So I can stretch my imagination to what it must be like for families who suffer sleep deprivation for months, years even. I understand why it can lead to postnatal depression and the break down of marital relationships.

So if you're at your wits end with sleep deprivation, using some kind of baby sleep training method, will help to improve things. But this inevitably means a little crying because you are changing habits, and that's not easy for any of us! Research and experience tells us that controlled crying or gradual withdrawal techniques work. What is key when using these techniques is that you respond to your baby's cries. As Leach says, this doesn't mean giving your baby what he wants when he is crying, it just means responding as a caring parent would.

If you're trying to teach your baby to fall asleep from awake by himself, and he has never done this before, then he might cry. If it's a proper cry (and not a grizzle), go ahead and reassure him of your support, but then put him back in his cot while he is awake so that he can try again to fall asleep by himself. Yes, he may protest, cry, scream even. And you can reassure him again, until he finally figures out how to get to sleep without your help.

As parents, I guess we're all just muddling through, aiming to get it right and wanting to do the best for our children. The choices we make are part of a bigger picture, created by our unique circumstances, family and baby. Add a touch of common sense and a lot of love and it's hard to go too wrong.

Nine Steps to Wean Your Baby Off Night Feeding

If your baby is over six months, eating three solid meals a day and still feeding at night, here are some tips to wean your baby off night feeds.

1- It's important to make sure your baby is getting enough food and milk in the day for her age and weight or she will continue to need a feed at night.

2 - Ensure your baby is getting enough day time sleep and napping well so you can be sure she isn't overtired at bedtime. An overtired baby may wake during the night and need your help to fall back to sleep. All the sleep training in the world won't be able to fix this.

3- Can she settle herself? It's important your baby is able to settle herself at nap time and bedtime. If she won't self settle you need to address the bed and naptime routines so that she knows when it's time for sleep, and not time for milk or play! Make a routine that works for you but which is consistent and predictable so baby knows what happens next. A baby comforter will help your baby to adapt to new sleep routines.

4- Does she feel safe? Creating a comforting, familiar, dark environment for your baby to sleep in is an important first step so that she always feels secure in her cot. If she still doesn't settle alone you may need to look at sleep training techniques, as she is likely to continue to wake in the night if she can't settle herself. Soothing music can help.

5 - Once you have established that your baby isn't hungry and taught her to self settle in a familiar environment she may stop waking at night within a few days.

6 - For a baby of 6 months or less, try introducing a last feed at 10:00pm. You should be able to do this while your baby is still asleep and this will help her to go for longer - hopefully until morning!

7 - If your baby is still waking at night you need to eliminate one night feed at a time. Start by delaying the feed when she initially wakes to see if she will settle alone. If she doesn't settle you can go in and comfort her whilst she is still in her cot. If your baby has a dummy you can offer that instead. Tell her it is sleep time, not milk time. Feed her next time she wakes and keep doing this every night, pushing it on a little at a time. Be careful you don't undo your work by going backwards! Over time the feed you are trying to eliminate will coincide with the next feed. Keep doing this with all night feeds until it becomes the first morning feed.

8 - If you find this very difficult, or if your baby becomes very upset, perhaps your partner could help? Sometimes dad going in makes things easier, sometimes not. It is often a case of trial and error.

9 - Maintain the late night feed (between 10 and 11pm) until your baby is between 7 and 9 months. Then start weaning your baby off this feed too. Some babies just do it themselves by taking so little milk that it is no longer worth your while giving it to them!

These key things, if consistently followed, will let your baby know that they need to sleep at night. If she does continue to wake during the night it may be worth trying sleep training techniques. As always, there is no hard and fast rule about what will work for you and your baby so it is best to read about different techniques before deciding what may work best.

What Is a Sleep Regression?

This is what a typical sleep regression looks like:

Your baby goes from sleeping through the night, to suddenly waking several times a night. They can't fall asleep, or stay asleep. They fight naps, bedtime, and wake frequently at night, often crying. Your baby is clingy, cranky and super needy during the day. You have ruled out illness, teething, and it's way longer than a few day growth spurt.

A sleep regression most commonly presents itself at around 4 months, 9 months, and 12 months. This is around the time that your baby is going through some major milestones: rolling, sitting, standing crawling, walking etc. What's actually happening with your baby is pretty interesting. Your baby is going through tremendous cognitive development. They are learning new skills and are practicing them in their head. Over and over, until they finally master the skill, which usually then terminates the regression. Your baby's brain during this time is in overdrive. Try to imagine for a minute what you feel like the night before a big event like going away on a vacation, or the night before your wedding. You stay up all night thinking about everything, making sure you don't forget anything. You toss and turn, and keep looking at the clock.

It keeps getting later and later and no matter what you do, you can't turn off your thoughts and just fall asleep. You start to get angry which makes it even harder to fall asleep. At this point you just want to scream! The next day you are over tired, cranky and just want to crawl back into your bed. This is exactly what's going on with your baby. Your baby can't turn off the brain work. She tries to soothe herself to sleep like she always did, but that doesn't seem to work. She often wakes up crying and screaming for your help, because she can't do it on her own. Your baby becomes overtired from all of this interrupted sleep, and ends up being cranky all day long.

So what do you do?

1.) Extra comfort during this time. Extra hugs and kisses. Try your best to settle your baby.

2.) Don't let your baby cry. Respond to her need.

3.) Pull out your bag of tricks (most of which you probably used when your baby was newborn). White noise, bouncer, binky, "lovie", whatever it takes to get your baby to sleep. You both need sleep, otherwise you will find it very difficult to make it through several week of this.

4.) Remember a sleep regression doesn't last forever, on average 2-6 weeks. Keep reminding yourself that this will pass, and your life will be back to normal soon.

5.) Sometimes there's not much you can do, but just tough it out. Stay strong, don't get frustrated, and take naps during the day to be handle the rough night

I have been through this and it's not pretty. My baby went from sleeping 12 hours to suddenly waking several times a night. I was so confused and frustrated, until my Pediatrician told me about the regression. Made total sense to me once it was explained. Brianna's sleep regression only last 2 weeks. I thought to myself "I have been through months of not sleeping, I can sure handle a couple weeks". So I just cuddled her more, responded right away, and even gave her extra feedings. I was so afraid that the extra feedings would be a major set back. I thought I would have to start sleep training all over again. But I knew she needed it during that time, and strongly believed that since she had already mastered the skills of falling asleep independently for several weeks, she would go back to that, once the regression was over. And guess what? That's exactly what happened. Once she worked out whatever she was working on in her little noggin, she immediately went back to sleeping 12 hours a night.

I look at sleep regression like when you first bring your baby home from the hospital. Anything goes at that point, anything she needs you provide. No set rules. So that the both of you get some sleep, otherwise you'll slowly start to lose your sanity. Don't be afraid that your going to have to start sleep training all over. Like I said, once your baby already has those skills, the most that you'll have to do is remind her, not start all over.

Why Babies Wake Up Crying

Many parents often wonder why their baby wakes up from sleep crying. Babies can typically wake up crying when they are hungry, because they are wet or dirty, or to have their sleep association recreated (such as replacing a pacifier), but this article is to discuss what it possibly means when your baby wakes up crying from a nap or in the morning when it seems like they are "done sleeping."

Current information and research indicates that there does not seem to be any definitive reason as to why babies cry when they wake up, but we do know it is normal for them to cry between sleep cycles. In the majority of cases, when a baby wakes up crying, it means he is not done sleeping. Sometimes a baby may have awakened in between sleep cycles and had trouble getting back to sleep for the next sleep cycle. Some babies have a much easier time going into the next sleep cycle and may just whimper a bit between sleep cycles.

Often, it is best if you not to run in at the slightest whimper because crying is normal and expected between sleep cycles. Babies might not cry every sleep cycle but there are some who do. You do not need to let your baby "cry-it-out", but for most parents any amount of crying feels a lot longer than it is. Many parents inadvertently find out that their baby just needed some time to resettle themselves when they cannot get to baby right away and when they do enter baby's room after a minute or two of crying, they find that baby has gone back to sleep. This is a prime indication that had the parent entered the room any earlier then they would have disturbed their baby's nap or sleep cycle.

Allow yourself the time to get to know and understand your baby's sleep cycles, sleep schedule and waking patterns. There are some babies who will wake up crying as part of their normal wake up routine and for others you will need to determine if your baby is simply resettling back into another sleep cycle. Until you have worked towards nap or sleep training with your baby as a way to help your baby learn to sleep through the night, try giving baby three to five minutes to resettle back to sleep without your help. Not only does this help baby to get the amount of sleep he needs but it can help him learn how to fall back asleep without creating a sleep association habit.

Creating Good Sleep Habits in Babies

Sleep is one of the most sought after things for a new parent. As every parent knows, the early days can be really difficult, as babies are up every few hours in the night looking for a feed. Some babies sleep really well from the outset, but these children are rare indeed. The majority of parents experience difficulties with sleep deprivation, and unfortunately for some, this can last well into the toddler years and beyond.

So how do you create a better sleeping environment for your baby? There are lots of things you can do to help create the right sleep associations and avoid the bad ones. A sleep association is essentially what the baby associates with going to sleep - in other words it is a learned response. Babies are clever because they get to know these associations by repetition - the more you do a certain behaviour before they sleep, the more they associate that behaviour with sleep itself. So for example, if you always bath the baby before bedtime, they will get to know in time that bathtime signals sleep time.

The trick is to create sleep associations which work without reliance on the parent to help the child to sleep, Some examples of poor sleep associations includes:

- ➤ Rocking baby to sleep
- ➤ Holding baby to sleep
- ➤ Patting/stroking baby
- ➤ Nursing or feeding baby to sleep
- ➤ Use of a dummy

Why are these poor sleep associations? Because they work by allowing the baby to rely on either you or a pacifier to help them sleep. This creates long-term problems because each time your child wakes at night, they will require your assistance to help put them back to sleep. Imagine you always rock baby to sleep. As wonderfully nurturing as it seems, what will you do when the child gets older and heavier and puts pressure on your back because you are struggling to rock your toddler to sleep - something that can take an hour or so in some cases?

The best solution is creating sleep associations that do NOT rely on you to help them sleep. These can include:

- ➤ Creating a routine
- ➤ Winding down
- ➤ Dimming the lights and speaking softly
- ➤ Placing tired baby in cot in the dark and calming them down by speaking softly and not picking them up
- ➤ Differentiating between night and day
- ➤ Removing the dummy before baby falls asleep
- ➤ Never allowing baby to sleep in your arms
- ➤ Always let baby sleep in the cot

These are just some suggestions, but there are many other things you can and should do to improve sleep. If you stick to your guns, you should see an improvement in sleep patterns within a week, and certainly within two weeks. With older children, you may need to resort to sleep training methods to help them sleep soundly.

Learning the correct behaviour takes time, but the above mentioned ideas are the best way to help a newborn learn the correct sleep habits that will set them up for a lifetime.

The Truth Behind the Back Sleep Position For Infants

The present threat of Sudden Infant Death Syndrome (SIDS) among infants has created a stir not only to mothers, but to medical experts as well. Over the years, modern science have been looking for better sleeping position that can prevent such tragedy.

Among babies, sleeping on one's back is recommended as opposed to sleeping on one's stomach. It has been a popular myth that when babies are allowed to sleep on their backs, they are most likely to choke. This is actually not the case. Most babies do vomit or spit during sleep. When this happens, some believed that babies are prone to choking when they are in a back sleep position. The truth is - babies involuntarily swallow any fluid they produce while in sleep. Doctors state that there has been no instance where such incidents were increased with such sleeping position.

A distinguished medical organization, the American Academy of Pediatrics, recommended infants to sleep on their backs. Medical experts attest that the back sleep position can decrease the risk of SIDS. Modern research shows that the chances of acquiring SIDS among children were lowered dramatically by almost 40% each year if such sleeping position was implemented. It is actually beneficial for babies if they are in this position as they can easily move their arms and legs.

Babies who are 2- 4 months old are likely to shift positions, put them back to the back sleep position by carefully rolling them over. Another option is to carefully swaddle them in a comfortable blanket to prevent them from sleeping on their stomach. You can also get one of those special swaddling blankets available in the market.

At first, your babies may find it uncomfortable to sleep on their backs because they naturally sleep on their stomachs. It would be the parents' or the guardians' responsibilities to train them in the back sleep position. With enough practice, they would eventually make it a sleeping habit. When training your babies, remember to remind your relatives or babysitters who might put your child into sleep in case of your absence.

Common Sleep Busters

The most common occurrence that parents experience is a baby waking up several times at night. This is almost always due to some type of attachment or dependency on something or someone. Babies are smarter than we may think, and can form habits very quickly and easily. By complying with their requests once or twice, parents help dependency habits to become entrenched and can actually make their children's sleep issues worse.

As a parent, you want to provide for all of your baby's needs - emotionally, developmentally and physically - and you don't want your baby to feel abandoned or unloved... ever! At the same time, however, it is important to help him to develop healthy sleep habits, so that he can grow properly and so that you will have the energy and patience to take care of him during the day.

"The Transfer"

Many parents make the mistake of putting their baby to sleep in one setting, and then transferring him to another (stroller to crib, mommy's arms to stroller, etc.). This can be exhausting for the parents and very confusing for a baby. It becomes an all-night merry-go-round of getting your baby to sleep in one place and then transferring him to where you'd like him to sleep for the remainder of the night,

99

only to have him wake up - causing you to begin your song-and-dance all over again. The key is to teach your baby both how to fall asleep and how to stay asleep on his own - so that you can both sleep better.

Falling Asleep at the Breast or Bottle

It is natural for a newborn to simply fall asleep while sucking at the breast, bottle or pacifier. However, when a baby becomes accustomed to falling asleep in this way, an association with sucking and falling asleep is produced. Often parents of older babies with sleep problems are still struggling with this association! By learning how to get rid of this association, you will enable your baby to fall asleep on his own, while still having the comfort of the breast, bottle or pacifier.

Waking for Night-Time Feedings

As mentioned above, newborns and smaller babies cannot go for long stretches at night without a feeding. Older babies who are receiving the proper nutrition and dietary intake during the day, however, should be able to sleep well through the night (assuming they are sleeping and eating properly during the day as well). By learning what your baby needs and when he needs it, you will be able to help him get better, fuller sleep. For example, a baby who snacks several times a night will never be satisfied and will wake up more often than a baby who simply has one solid, hearty feeding in the night. Also, babies often whimper or cry at night simply because they are coming in and out of different sleep rhythms. Therefore, it is crucial to learn your baby's nighttime sounds in order to better differentiate whether he is actually waking due to hunger, or when he is simply transitioning into various rhythms in his sleep.

Rocking to Sleep, Holding etc.

When you continually rock or hold your child to sleep, you may not realize that you are fostering this habit, since he will be unable to naturally acquire the proper tools to calm himself when he needs to.

A baby who does not know how to sleep on his own will only continue to be dependent on an outside source and will never have the restful sleep he needs in order to properly develop and function throughout the day.

NOTE: It is always important to address any medical concerns before making any significant changes in your child's sleep habits.

The most important factor to keep in mind, however, is that a problem only exists when you feel it does, and as the parent of your baby you know what is best. Only you can determine when to implement changes to tackle your baby's sleep challenges as any plan of action will only be successful when you are ready for it.

Babies and Sleeping - What Parents Forget

Babies are tender and innocent. With all the stress and pressure faced by a new parent, it is very easy to forget this. Due to a painstakingly laborious job of childcare, many parents get tired and began neglecting the most important safety precautions.

Experts recommend not giving juice or a milk formula before bedtime. Make sure that you take the bottle away, before they sleep otherwise it will cause baby bottle tooth decay. If the baby gets on sleep with a bottle in its mouth then water is a very safe choice. Don't give your baby a solid food before he is at least six months old. Doctors always ask mothers to breast feed in the first months. A mother's milk is designed by nature to provide every ingredient that the child will initially need.

A solid food in the first six months will only put the baby at the mercy of stomach virus. A bad stomach means a bad night sleep. Very young babies should not have any kind of toys in their cribs. Toys can easily result in suffocation. Yes! Much older babies can have toys in the crib bit just make sure that the toys don't disturb your child. One or two favorite toys will do the trick.

101

Never threaten your child to go to bed. Bedtime should serve to relax the nerves. Many parents force their kids to the bed which ultimately leads to bad bedtime memories. Children should think of a bed time as a time to rest and have good dreams, not the opposite. Too many chocolates and soda may contain enough dose of caffeine to seriously hamper any sleep pattern, among children. Often, Pediatrics fail to explain the affects of watching TV before a bed time. Just remember, it is the single most notorious reason for sleep disorders.

Baby Temperament and Sleep Series

During this series, we have reviewed 9 temperament traits that make up all of our personalities and seen how they might affect the way you help your baby or toddler sleep better. I've grouped some of the temperaments together to give you some ideas on helping your baby or toddler sleep better.

Adaptable, Regular, and Positive First Reaction

If your baby or toddler is adaptable, she is probably a little more easy-going than other babies. If she skips a nap, she might not get cranky and will take it in stride. Her regularity makes it easy to plan play dates around her nap schedule and potty training might be really easy if she pees and poops at the same time every day. It might even be easier to master elimination communication, where you can gradually reduce the number of diapers you use for your baby by learning their rhythms and signs before they "go". If your baby or toddler also typically has a positive first reaction to a new person, food, event or change to routine, she will likely not skip a beat to many changes in her sleep routine at once.

A baby with these temperament traits will likely respond well to a nudge from mom and dad when it comes to solving her sleep problems or breaking sleep associations. It will likely be a lot easier than you think to break some habits and get on a good routine and sleep schedule with your baby and all you need is a little confidence, time, and patience. All you have to do is take the first step and try.

Sensitive, Perceptive, and Adaptable

If your baby is sensitive, he will be more apt to wake up from noises, care more about being hot or cold, and be in tune with your own emotions or stress. Your baby might also notice a lot more around him and things might keep him awake by catching his attention if he is perceptive.

When it comes to sleep, combining sensitivity and perceptive-ness, your baby might be a little more "high maintenance" than our adaptable and regular counter parts above, but if he is also adaptable, he might be able to change his sleeping habits fairly easily. You may just need to go through extra steps helping him sleep through noise, be comfortable (especially during things like teething), and make sure his room is dark enough that it will not distract him too much from the task at hand (sleeping). Some of his other temperament traits will be a factor in terms of how easy or difficult it will be to break problematic sleep associations.

Intense, Persistent, and Energetic

Probably one of the most difficult temperament traits is the intense child. She does not whimper or fuss, she wails and SCREAMS! When she's happy, she's HAPPY but when she's not WATCH OUT! She will let you know loudly how she feels about something. Combine this trait with her persistence and you can have fairly long and loud temper tantrums when she doesn't get that cookie or toy in the store.

When it comes to sleep, the intense and persistent baby or toddler will probably be much more challenging to help learn to sleep. Disclaimer:

103

I could be partial to saying that because my eldest son, who inspired this site, is both intense and persistent, of course. He also has a lot of energy. This combination of temperament traits are most likely a part of the babies you hear "cry all night" if the parents let them. My son did not, so I know there are more intense and more persistent babies out there. Cry it out is not the only option for these babies, either. It highly depends on your baby and your own temperament, too.

These are arbitrary temperament trait combinations I put together and obviously this list is not exhaustive (doing the math because I'm a nerd, it's 512 combinations if we assumed a trait is on or off, which obviously is not true so chew on that for awhile and just think how long that article would be!). Although you believe your baby will be the hardest there is, the chances are actually small and you might really be surprised how small a nudge you might have to give your baby to encourage her to sleep on her own. I talk to MANY parents who are pleasantly surprised how much "easier" it was than they originally thought it would be.

Taking the first step, making a "sleep coaching" plan, to help your child sleep is the hardest part, especially when the "easy" answers haven't worked for you in the past when that neighbor says "I just put her down awake and she went to sleep". Not so easy for all of us. Some parents are also so judgmental about the method some parents choose to help their child sleep, but unless you have "that" temperament kid, you really don't know what that other person might be going through and since all babies are a unique combination of these traits, you won't ever have someone else be able to walk in your shoes or vice versa. Don't be so quick to say what you think you'd do in the same situation. Even if you have a tough sleeper, how YOU react to sleep deprivation will be different.

While many feel the only choice is sleep deprivation or cry it out, there is A LOT in between, depending on your baby's temperament. Don't let sleep deprivation be the choice you make. You owe it to

104

yourself and your baby or toddler to get the rest you both need to function at your optimum!

CHAPTER FIVE

Toddler Sleeping Behavior

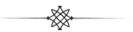

W hat better way for a family to help their toddler achieve independence than by encouraging him to learn to sleep alone? Sleep provides a natural opportunity to foster the separation process, because at least eight hours every day of the year a toddler does it. While many blogs offer helpful tips, I believe that the key to understanding your child's bedtime habits is viewing them as issues of separation.

Sleep is a problem for toddlers precisely because it coincides with their developmental task of becoming separate from you. And of course, nothing during this age comes easily. Sleeping alone in a room without a mother or father can bring out all a toddlers anxieties about being on his own.

It's understandable that sleep-deprived parents want their child's bedtime issues resolved immediately. When parents reach the point where they can't stand another night of exhaustion, it can be hard to be patient. But remember that a toddler will not become a good sleeper overnight. There are suggestions that should help in the ups and downs of sleep, but they are not a total cure for problems.

Separation is a slow process affected by how parents react to their toddler's growing independence. For instance, do you feel lonely or worried when your child isn't right next to you? Like toilet training and giving up bottles or pacifiers, a child learns how to be a good sleeper when she feels that her parents have faith in her ability to become one.

Additionally, what happens during a toddler's day is going to affect his night. If he had a fight with his friend or if he has a new baby-sitter, he very well might spend half the night calling out for his parents. Or if he didn't get enough hugs and cuddles because his parents were out most of the day, he might wake to get them. Some children will never become long sleepers no matter what their mother and father do. While many toddlers sleep between twelve and fourteen hours daily, others do quite well on eight to ten hours.

Every family must decide on what sleeping arrangements are best suited to their own beliefs and cultural standards. Do you think a baby should stay in her parents' room until she is one? Or do you think a three-month-old should be sleeping in her crib in her own room? Were you brought up sharing a room with siblings? Did your parents not mind you spending part of the night in bed with them? Or were you one of those children who always enjoyed cuddling up under your blanket with your teddy bear in your own bed?

It may be hard to believe when your toddler cries out for you at 3 A.M., but sleep can be another source of pleasure, solace, and joy for your toddler just as playing, eating, running, and talking can be.

Bedding Comfort for Your Baby

Your baby is your life... the comfort, care and feeding of your child consumes much of your day and evening existence. There is so much to know, to be aware of, that even with all of the expert advice from family and friends, there's still a great deal to be learned, either through study of various resources, or through the daily experience of raising your child.

Most mothers and fathers would say the comfort of their baby is one of their prime concerns. Comfort is the baby's world, from the temperature in the home, their diapers, their cleanliness, their food and drink, their clothing and their baby bedding. All of these elements should be designed to ensure the safety and health of the child and to make their small world a happy and enjoyable place within which to grow.

Afternoon naps, breast-feeding, and nighttime sleep require coverings to keep the baby warm. These coverings must be soft enough to ensure a warm environment, resilient enough to withstand stains, and secure enough to prevent accidents. There are a number of elements to the selection of appropriate baby and crib bedding. Thankfully, there are a number of baby bedding sets now available that assist with the continual drain on your financial resources to ensure your baby's health.

When purchasing baby bed linens, highly advisable is to purchase four top and four bottom sheets. These can be of the fitted or flat varieties and are uniform in size. However, if you have a crib, cot, cot bed or Moses basket, sheet sizes differ. Make certain you know the size you need before you shop.

Try to obtain a minimum of four, high-quality blankets. Cold nights are not a pleasant reality for a baby. The best combinations for a baby blanket are those that offer breathability and warmth, such as cotton cellular blankets and fleece.

A sleeping bag is also a good alternative, but you'll need at least two of them. Babies have a tendency to wriggle at night. This can result in sheets and blankets being tossed all over the crib or bed, leaving the youngster cold. A sleeping bag ensures their comfort while restricting their movement. Plus, you won't need to purchase a top sheet or blanket.

If your child is at least one year old, you can obtain pillows and duvets. The duvet cover set and pillow are comfortable for your child and also assist in supporting his or her attempts to sit up. Be certain to remove cot bumpers if your child is at the sitting up stage.

For the newborn baby, crib bedding is what needs to be obtained. Again, the sizes are different than would be considered for a baby bed, and the baby's comfort must remain the parents' prime concern.

If you are traveling with your child, perhaps to see grandma and grandpa or a distant aunt or uncle, to include them in the joyful world of your child's existence, other considerations must be made for your baby's needs. There are now services that will ship all of your baby's needs to a specified address. This means Mom and Dad don't have to pack as though they are going on a safari with their child's food, diaper, and formula needs. Everything they require will be awaiting them when they reach their destination, whether a private home or a hotel room.

Baby-proofing the location where you will stay is another important element to keep in mind. From a cover clamp toilet lock to a sound monitor, a bi-fold door lock to cabinet slide locks, and those all important rail nets for indoor balconies or outdoor decks, all should be considered as critical to your baby or child's safety at your temporary location. Make certain you have information at hand as to where your child will be sleeping and either pack, or have delivered, the required baby or crib bedding to ensure his or her comfort.

Baby and crib bedding is one of those elements that cannot be overlooked. These items are critical to your continued success in rearing your baby in safety and comfort.

Coping with Infant Sleep Disorders

As an adult, it's likely that you suffer from insomnia at least occasionally. Unfortunately, even though it seems like babies sleep a lot, babies as well as adults can have sleep problems, too. Sometimes, they can morph over from the occasional disturbance to an actual sleep disorder.

If this happens, the first thing you need to do is to get your child to a doctor so that the baby can be properly diagnosed. Of course, infants sleep a lot when very small and in fact spend most of their early weeks eating and sleeping. As they grow, they'll spend more and more time awake. For the first few weeks, however, for the most part, the baby won't be doing much other than eating, sleeping and soiling diapers.

As children get older, of course, it becomes much more exciting to stay awake than it does to go to sleep. Many young children have the idea that they are "missing something" every time they go to sleep. Adults simply have endless fun when they're awake, while the child is stuck with boring old sleep. Of course, this isn't true, but this is something that children go through to at least some extent for the most part.

The best way to make sure children go to bed without much trouble is to establish a regular routine. Follow the routine every night. For example, perhaps just after dinner, it's time for bath. Once the child is in pajamas and ready for bed, some quiet playtime with toys in his or her room is to follow, followed by bedtime story, tucking in with stuffed animals or favorite blanket, and lights out.

Most children also go through periods when they experience nightmares or "the monster under the bed." Again, this is usually pretty normal. Because young children sleep comparatively more than adults do as well and the line between imagination and reality is necessarily blurred at that age, sometimes sleep and wake patterns are much closer together for them, especially at night, so they may be "dreaming awake" for some of what the experience. Again, if this is true, simply being soothing and reassuring, while making sure that the child knows he or she needs to stay in bed, is the best way to handle this. (Of course, older children are very, very good about getting "spooky" monsters to delay bed times and other undesirable events, so of course, smart parents are aware of this and make sure these types of monsters are put in their places.)

For some babies just home from the hospital, especially if premature, they may suffer from sleep apnea. The parents who bring these infants home are required to go through courses for CPR, and many are also trained in the use of monitors for children so that they can be instantly alerted if babies stop breathing. This is a common cause for the disorder known as crib death, and such babies will likely be put on monitors so that parents will be alerted immediately if the baby should stop breathing. Simply nudging the baby or rubbing his or her back is usually enough to get these little ones who just aren't quite old enough to know better to breathe on their own again.

By the time children are about six months old, the most acute danger for death has passed, with two years generally considered a safe age for no longer being at risk for this disorder. Your doctor will be able to tell you when your child no longer needs to be monitored for sleep apnea.

Learn to Blanket Train Your Baby

When you have a baby, sometimes all you need are some moments of silence. Especially when that silence is required in some situations like when you are in a plane, at the church or maybe in a bus. You can teach your baby to be silent in those particular situations, by blanket training him. I will show you in this article a method that has done wonders for a lot of mothers that now have no trouble with their baby's crying.

Here are the steps that you have to follow

First you have to choose a baby blanket that should be pretty comfortable. I recommend that the same baby blanket will be used for every training session. If you do that, he will develop a reflex and when he will see that particular blanket, will know that it is his quiet time. Now that you have chosen the blanket, some baby toys are required; toys that your baby loves would be great, but make sure that they are silent toys, such as plush teddy bears. You should have different ones, because the baby might get bored with the same toy, and also you will be using these toys only during training sessions.

Blanket training should begin at an early age. The baby should spend each day on the blanket a couple of hours. But when he will grow older, the blanket time should decrease, because babies get bored very fast. Also, I think that more important for his health is for the baby to take walks and discover new things then sitting all day long on a blanket, isn't it? You can try putting him to sleep on the blanket too, by singing or talking to him.

This training method should be repeated for a long period of time. Remember that the baby can't understand what you want him to do at a very early age, so you will need to be patient with him. He will want to crawl from the blanket when he will be able to do it. Put him back on the blanket and let him know that what he did was wrong and in time he will understand what you want from him.

Tips about baby Blanket Training

Be consistent. That is the only way that results will show. Your baby won't learn to stay still on the blanket when you want him to do over night, so be patient.

A one year old baby is more difficult to train then a few months old one, so start the blanket training at an early age.

Results may vary depending on the baby's personality.

Baby Tracker - Keeping Track of What Is Normal and What Is Not

You can use baby tracker software to track how well your baby's days go. Such software allows you to track feeding, diapers, growth, sleep, health, medicines, activities, and many other aspects of your baby's daily routine. This software provides you with the information you need to see how well things are going. More than one authorized user can see the information for each baby. That means parents, the baby sitter, daycare and anyone else can see what is going on. It is a good way to keep track of what is happening when there is more than one caregiver involved.

Why should you use baby tracker software to monitor your baby's feeding? Baby's often show the first signs of problems when their feeding starts changing. One non-normal feeding is not an indication of a problem. However, if your baby shows a series of non-normal feedings, it could be a sign of trouble. This software also helps you find when your baby begins to feed more. Babies go through growth spurts. Your baby may hit a time when their feeding needs increase. This software will help you track it and show it to your pediatrician. That information is invaluable when problems arise.

Baby tracker software also helps you monitor diaper changes. It helps to track when you last changed the diapers. It helps you identify your baby's normal patterns. It also helps you spot when your baby's patterns get off track. The software tracks whether the diaper was wet or contained stool. It allows you to track what the texture and color of the stool was. When potty training, this information can be just what you need in order to obtain the best results. It also helps you track diaper use to let you know when you need to stock up on more.

You can track your baby's sleeping patterns with baby tracker software as well. Sleep is a big part of any baby's day. It is important to track your baby's normal sleep patterns to help you keep track of what is normal and what is not. You can also find out where your baby's sleep the best. You can get the information in a variety of forms. You can take this information to your pediatrician. You can print it out to show to the babysitter. All of the different forms of information you track allows you to keep track of how well your baby progresses and when abnormal things come up.

Massage Is Good for Babies Too

As exciting as it may seem, having a newborn is certainly not a walk in the park. Dealing with erratic feeding schedules, disturbances in the sleeping pattern, and constant dealings with unexplained crying may sometimes just too much to be deal with. All of these spell stress for the parents, especially for the new ones. However, before you fuss and lose control, be informed that there is one modest way to totally relax your babies! Parents and soon-to-be-parents may delight now with the benefits that infant massage can bring.

Massage as a technique that utilizes different levels of touch and kinesthetic stimulation, can bring about advantages both for the mother and the babies, says several studies. Indeed, infant massage goes beyond from simply relaxing your babies and putting them to sleep. Through gentle and rhythmic strokes-tender manipulation of your baby's head, face, chest, tummy, legs, and feet-a gentle rubdown will not only benefit your babies but will also promote parent-to-child attachment.

So, what are the other benefits of massage? According to a study conducted by the researchers from Warwick Medical School and the Institute of Education at the University of Warwick, parents can help promote good sleep quality among their infants by provisioning a tender massage. Basing on the data gathered among 598 subjects, infants who received massage therapy seemed more relaxed when compared to those who are in the control group. This relaxed state, according to the study, can be attributed to the lower levels of cortisol, a stress hormone, present in the intervention group.

Moreover, infant massage has also been known to promote the baby's overall physical and psychosocial development. Physiologically speaking, massage can help babies with digestive difficulties. Experts recommend massage therapy for babies, who are experiencing colic, as it may help to remove spasms in the colon. Massage is also generally good in relieving elimination problems such as constipation and in expelling gas. In addition, gentle stimulation of your babies can also help to improve immune system, promote muscle development, ease nasal congestion and reduce teething pains. Aside from that, it will also improve the hormonal, respiration, circulation, and nervous system functions.

On the other hand, the advantages of massage surpass not only the physical aspect but also the psychosocial aspect as well. Massage in babies connotes a deeper meaning; it implies communication between the baby and its primary caregiver. Through sensory stimulation, the baby becomes more alert and receptive to the mother's touch. In this manner, both the parents and the baby can engage in a reciprocal and gratifying interaction. Massage promotes bonding, making the baby feel secured and loved, and in return, the mother feels empowered knowing that she can respond readily to her baby's cues thus making her feel confident about her parenting skills.

The benefits of massage can be credited to the fact that physical touch is the first type of communication an infant receives, and among the basic senses, touch is the most developed at birth. With a gentle rubdown, parent and child bonding is made easier. Remember, you are not the only one who needs a comforting massage, babies do, too.

Baby Care Tips Every Mother Needs to Know

Baby care is something you never need to worry about. Only you need to learn a few tricks on how to feed the baby, how to get him to sleep and how to sooth him if he starts crying. Once you get a bit of training on these topics you never need to think much about it. The most important part is how to feed your little bundle of joy. If you are going to breast feed your baby, just follow the instructions you get while you are in the hospital.

When you come home, if your baby refuses to feed himself with breast milk, meet the nurse who trained you on breast feeding and ask her for advice. There are a few reasons for a baby to refuse suckling the breast of his mother.

The next most difficult thing you will encounter is the changing of diapers. However, the modern diapers are easier to manage no matter whether they are disposable ones or reusable ones made out of cloth. The most important thing with changing diapers of a baby is to have your diapers, wipes and ointments ready at hand when you are going to change them. There are many resources from where you could learn the proper procedure of changing diapers in case you come across a problem situation.

Bathing the baby is the next tough job on which you need to train yourself. Bathing time is enjoyable for both your baby and yourself. The first thing is to have all the supplies ready. Remember to talk to your baby while you bath him. Babies like this interaction.

You may use your regular bathtub, a baby bathtub or a container to bathe the baby. Keep the water temperature to 100°F. Most mothers feel the water with their wrists. Also bathe your baby in a room that is not cold.

When you bathe the baby wash her hair first and then come down. Diaper area is the last to wash. Sometimes soap may not be necessary on the delicate skin of your baby. Once the bathing is over, wrap him in a towel and do the wiping also with the same towel.

Once your baby is dry, dress him and let someone else hold him until you clean your bathroom. If not you might have to feed him and put him to sleep before doing so. It is not a good idea to leave him alone and do the clean up.

CHAPTER SIX

How To Make Sure A Baby Crib Is Safe

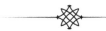

Investing in a good baby crib is necessary for the safety and comfort of your child. If you are expecting a new addition to your family, you will need to be sure you have a safe haven ready for your child's arrival. A good baby crib will prevent accidents and make you feel good about putting your child down for a nap. You should feel confident in your choice for years to come. A good baby crib can be used with multiple babies if you choose to have a lot of children.

The bedding you select can go with the decor you have chosen for your nursery. It should be easy to clean and flame retardant. It should not be too thick or heavy, so a child may not suffocate under it. Be sure to stock up on spare blankets, linings and mattress covers. You will need to be able to wash the bedding frequently, as much as every day if your child gets sick. There should be no zippers, beads, buttons, or any other ornaments that a child might choke on. Simple cribs are sometimes best. You will not need a lot of decorations or stuffed animals in the very beginning of your son or daughter's life.

One of the best things you can do for your child is to buy convertible baby cribs. These will follow your child through a few stages of life until he or she is finally ready for a big bed. Once the child is becoming old enough to walk, you will be able to convert the crib into a small bed, most likely by removing a side. If you trust the young child to stay in bed, you can start them early with this crib. But if you are afraid they will get into messes during the night, you can leave it in a crib setting on some nights or naps. A child that is being toilet trained should be allowed to get out of their bed during the night to use the bathroom to avoid nighttime accidents. Use your best judgement to decide whether or not you would need to buy a convertible crib.

A sleigh crib is one of the many styles you can choose from. Some of them are convertible, while others are vintage reproductions. The sleigh bed will be adorned with curves to make the baby crib look like a sleigh. These cribs are very stylish and might be the perfect thing for your decor. They receive a lot of compliments and will give your child good memories of sleeping in a beautiful wooden baby crib.

Baby Steps to a Healthy Life

We all want to live a healthy life. The choices we make decide on how healthy that life will be. There are certain people that take the "health thing" pretty seriously. They have made a commitment to be healthy and more fit. How do you live a healthier life?

Here are a few tips.

Wash your hands often for at least 20 to 30 seconds. A dose of preventions is better than an ounce of cure. Avoid certain behaviors such as smoking, excessive drinking of alcohol and eating excessively. That can dramatically improve your health all in it self. There are easy ways to get started being more healthy.

Strengthen Your Muscles

Muscles tend to weaken as we age. If you want to prevent a that from happening in a BIG way, you need to practice weight bearing exercises on a regular basis. Weight training increases lean muscles tissue. It also encourages bone Density. Bone density starts to decrease in our thirties but we can combat that with regular resistance training. Weight training also jump starts your metabolism and helps you to burn calories at a faster rate.

Go For A Walk

We are designed to be on the move. We started as hunters and gatherers on the move constantly. Walking actually triggers all of the bodies systems. digestion, stress relief, preparation for sleep, clarity of thinking. It is a free activity, It is easy, most everyone walks and you can get the exercise with out the wear and tear on your body.

Stop Drinking Soda

This is a big one. All of the processed sugars in these sugary drinks just makes you crave more. These drinks have contributed to the skyrocketing rates of obesity and type 2 diabetes. Diet soda is the worst because it tricks the brain with the sweetness but there are not any calories so the body is not satisfied and craves more. It is easy to put down 40 pounds of liquid calories a year by just having 2 glasses of milk, one glass of juice and one glass of wine a day. That is 200,750 calories a year the 40 pounds of liquid calories represents. Add soda to that and the calorie count could easily double along with the liquid calories consumed. These are all USELESS calories that do nothing but eat your teeth and add unwanted pounds.

Keep a Food Journal

You can double your weight loss by just writing down everything you eat. Doctors have found the more people wrote down what they ate the more weight they loss. We become aware of our habits when we go through the process of reflecting on what we eat. That is the only way to change a behavior, to become fully aware of it. There are online food journal sights that can make it easy or you can get yourself a cheap notebook and write it all down there. Make sure you include the time so you can see any patterns forming with they type of food and the time. Make sure to write how you felt at the time. Measure your hunger from 1 to 10, just that alone may keep you from putting that extra helping on your plate.

Relax, take a "Chill"

If you are a stressed out person, you are more vulnerable to colds and flu all winter long. When you get sick it will take longer to recover if you are a stressed out person. People that do not know how to relax gain more weight and get more illnesses than a person that has learned to "Chill". People that have learned to combat stress sometimes use exercise or specifically weight training to relieve it. Some find peace in music or humor. Other good ways to reduce stress are Tai Chi and Yoga.

Get Plenty Of Sleep

People really over look this factor. Sleep is one of the most important aspects of health. Without it hormone levels go "whacky" and you do not have the energy that you might have, you gain weight easily and you are moody. Do not put your self in the path of the flu this season. Not getting enough rest will make you more susceptible to what ever is going around. One thing that helps sleep is to have a routine and stick to it. No excitement late in the evening, a dark sleeping environment that is 50 to 60 degrees is best.

Eat Outside The Home Less Often

Eating out at restaurants just makes you loose control of what you are eating. Many times they get prepared foods and fail to really cook anything. many additives and preservatives are used in the foods and many meats are soaked in a "salt brine" to keep it from spoiling (salt is a preservative). Be careful about the foods you buy for home, Look at the label. Be aware of sodium levels and keep them as low as possible. Be a conscious eater.

Eat Whole Foods and Go Organic Where You Can

Any un-processed or un-refined with no added sugar, salt or fat. usually whole foods have a low glycemic index so they will not increase your blood sugar and insulin levels as quickly as processed foods. Eat wheat bread, stay away from french fries. Eat as many fresh fruits and vegetables as possible. Stay away from anything in a bag, box, or can.

Find Your Passion

What is Life without passion?

Life needs to have meaning or we are not fulfilled and that is not something that we enjoy. having a "higher purpose in life" can reduce the risk of death among older adults. Purpose is stimulating cognitively so the real truth is "use it or loose it", they have been saying it for years, now I believe it. Everyone needs to feel useful and have interests or what is life about.

Be As Social As Possible

 The reason that we are so social as human beings is that we re-create and in order to do that we need to communicate (although some of us do that better than others). In order to create a strong sense of social identity it is necessary to belong to social groups, clubs, teams or church is another option. Having this strong sense of social identity significantly reduces your chance of having a stroke, dementia, and even our yearly common illnesses such as the flu and a cold. Loneliness breeds both illness and early death.

Common Symptoms of an Unhappy Baby

 As a parent it can be difficult to detect development issues as your baby can't tell you if there is problem and where it hurts. Often there may be issues that you aren't even aware of, or people tell you is simply 'normal' for a baby.

Far to often I see babies who have dislocated shoulders or subluxated necks who are unable to feed on one breast or favouring sleeping on one side, yet their mothers are told it is normal. It is certainly not normal.

Some common symptoms of an unhappy baby that chiropractic may be able to help with are:

- Relentless crying
- Colic
- Favour turning head to one side
- Unable to attach properly to the breast for feeding/ difficulties with attachment during breast feeding
- Not sleeping for long periods
- Flattened skull or miss-shapen head
- Reflux
- Constipation.

These can all have serious implications on a baby's health and spinal and nervous system, and have serious consequences to their development. Therefore, it is very important to have your chiropractor check your baby as early as day one. I will often adjust babies on the day they come into the world (as well as mum and dad).

Let the Experts Help

Chiropractors are well trained to detect interferences to a baby's nervous system and apply gentle, delicate treatments to give them the best start in life. The pressure I apply to newborns is like checking a tomato to see how ripe it is. It is extremely gentle, safe and effective.

Recently there was a media story about the finding of the remains of the English King Richard III. The archaeologists who discovered the skeleton had a strong lead when they initially unearthed the remains - a distinctly bent spine, a clear indication of scoliosis, something historians reported King Richard suffered from. Had Richard been seeing a chiropractor from a young age, early detection of his scoliosis, followed by regular chiropractic treatment could have helped to correct the issue. He may not have had to endure the pain of scoliosis and all those hunchback jibes.

There is a saying 'so bent the twigs grows the tree', which means the earlier you begin correcting a problem the less likely it is to develop into something worse.

If you suspect there is an issue with your baby then please contact your local chiropractor and arrange to go in for a check, the chiropractor will make sure everything is functioning as it should.

What Are Sleep Issues That Affect Your Child?

Some of the most common concerns that parents of young children express are about sleep issues. It can be highly disruptive for the entire family when a child has problems going to sleep or wakes up many times during the night.

Disorders that affect sleep in children are not that much different than those occurring in adults, yet sleeping problems in children are far more common. It is considered a problem when a sleep pattern is causing disruptions in adolescent or toddler behavior.

Night terrors usually occur in children who are three to eight years old and happen approximately 90 minutes after falling to sleep. Your child may suddenly sit upright and scream, and be inconsolable. As frightening as they might be, rest assured that they usually go away on their own. Alleviating stress and ensuring that your child is getting enough rest is all that can be done to combat night terrors.

Sleepwalking and sleep talking can be another concern for parents and they should take steps to make balconies or stairs safe, since sleepwalkers can experience physical harm. Their bedroom should be on the first floor of the home, with the windows and doors firmly secured. Parents should keep interventions to a minimum as these sleep behaviors generally do not require any interference, except for safety. This disorder is usually outgrown by adolescence.

Bed wetting can cause serious sleep issues. It is considered to be one of the most prevalent and persistent causes of sleep problems. Kids who are developmentally behind from age one to three are more likely to still be wetting the bed at age six. It cannot be construed as an uncooperative child unwilling to toilet train or just simply unpleasant behavior after that point. This problem tends to run in families.

While colic is not a sleep problem on the surface, colicky infants appear to have a shorter duration of sleep. Colic is often the bane of a new parent's existence in that sleep problems may sometimes persist after the child has outgrown the colic. Strategies that parents developed to cope with the crying spells, like frequently holding the infant or car rides can interfere with the adaptation of normal sleep patterns.

Make sure to put your child to bed while they are still awake. This gives them a chance to learn how to fall asleep on their own and this will avoid many sleep issues. Keep in mind that just because your child has slept through the night a few times, this doesn't mean it will occur every night. Most babies don't sleep through the night on a consistent basis. Be aware that with each new milestone your child reaches, like when they start potty training, they may also resume waking in the night.

Smart Babies: 20 Easy Ways to Make Your Baby Smart

Some babies are naturally prone to be smart by genetics, while others are less apt to get the 'genius gene'. Of course, every parent hopes for the latter. However, as parents it is our duty to nurture and harness the full potential of our children from birth.

There are many misconceptions and old wives' tales when it comes to raising babies, but speaking from first-hand experience, there are a number of development milestones that a baby can reach much earlier than any expert's predictions. Most of these benchmarks are the result of positive and patient parenting, which is the underlying requirement for having a smart baby.

Yet, parents are often too busy, too tired and just too lazy (no offense) to take the time that is needed for a baby's early development. As a result, kids these days have a tough time at school compared to kids of only a generation or two ago. They use less of their imaginations and more technological stimulants, which have been proven in studies to make people less smart than those who read books or spend no time in front of the TV.

Other external culprits could include one or both parents being gone a lot, or having undesirable family environments such as homes where fighting, bickering or negatively yelling and reprimanding children takes place. Such an atmosphere is upsetting to a child; therefore they may become withdrawn and less excited about learning. They get less attention than a child who has both parents; or one who lives in a home that is emotionally happy.

Assuming the baby has none of these obstacles, there is no reason why he or she should be hindered by early intelligence growth. Babies as early as a few days old can begin learning and can understand words much sooner than they can speak.

Here are 20 ways to encourage early learning development for your baby:

1. Talk out everything you do or see with your baby. As you take the baby for a walk, point to flowers, birds and cars and say the word as

you show the baby what you are saying. The baby learns what these things are, as well as becoming more alert and aware of his environment.

2. Read books from day one. People laughed that I read books to my newborn, but by 6 - 7 months old, he was already able to turn the pages in anticipation of the rest of the book and could understand much of what the books were about based on the pictures and my daily explanations. He often dragged his favorite books to be read again, and again!

3. Index Cards. I cannot stress the value of these great 'toys'. Choose index cards that have a front and back - with the letter or number on one side and pictures that accompany that letter on the back. The baby will play with them and look forward to them. Don't worry about reading them in order, just pick one up occasionally and read it. Soon your baby will be doing the same. Make these cards fun and your baby will learn letters before you know it. Make fun games with the cards, such as spelling out his name.

4. Bring the baby everywhere. I know, getting bundled up and dressed can be a pain, but your baby soaks up these experiences and will look forward to it. He gets to meet people, see the world and watch others instead of just staring at his own living room every day. As well, some parents balk at the idea of traveling far away with an infant, but these experiences can be very mentally stimulating for him. We brought our baby to two NFL games already with thousands of people. He loved it! Getting used to crowds will help him develop socially.

5. Do things with the baby that you would normally do. Let him watch you brush your teeth, hair and get dressed. Although it may take longer for you to do these simple tasks, the baby will learn and watch everything you do. It makes teaching him easier and faster.

6. Avoid using TV (even kid's shows) as a babysitter. Some parents stick their kids in front of the TV because they are too tired or lazy to interact with them. The only programs your child should watch are specific educational DVDs, preferably one to accompany the index cards. My baby has been using them since approx. 2 months old and already says many words from this video. Parents who chime in and interact as the baby is watching will aid in his interest and learning.

7. Listen to music and sing and dance with baby. Our baby loves electronic and house music. Strange, yes. But the upbeat tempo and energetic style puts him in a great mood, as well as stimulating his mind. He has been interested in music since day one and we often choose low tempo techno songs to dance him to sleep. Babies love music, and just as versatile as the parents. Some may love Country music, house music, classical, orchestra or whatever the mother liked to listen to as the baby was growing in the womb.

8. Give your baby choices. Teach him colors by saying what color things are as you give it to him. "Yellow banana. Blue Ball. Which one do you want?" As the baby grabs the item, repeat the one he chooses back to him.

9. While pregnant, take prenatal vitamins. Intelligence begins in the womb, so take all-natural prenatal vitamins instead of prescribed or over-the-counter remedies from pharmacies. These can be stacked throughout the day. Your baby has a stronger chance of being smart from birth if he's had the proper supplementation throughout the duration of your pregnancy.

10. Let other people hold your baby. As long as the person is safe, doing this will help your baby learn about individuality. There is nothing more precious than a baby's assessment of another human. Babies do not have any prejudice, judgments or concern over whether someone is fat or thin, what they look like, or anything other than if

the person is 'fun' or not. Let people hold your baby and he will learn about the characteristics of human beings.

11. Stay happy, no matter what. Even when you have a bad day. As a parent, babies pick up on your energy. If you're in a bad mood, distressed, upset or angry, the baby will also become distressed. Always smile and make your baby feel good. Happier babies are smarter babies.

12. Use positive reinforcement. As soon as your baby does something you have taught him - no matter how insignificant it may be - make a big deal about it! Yell, "Good boy!" and repeatedly encourage your baby to make these efforts for your approval. Your baby will become more determined and happy to please you.

13. Let baby look in the mirror. Allow him to study his reflection and praise him while he does. "What a handsome boy... smart boy... cute boy...etc." Tell your baby he is great and that he can be anything he wants in life!

14. Let him touch things. Of course, there are some things you don't want your baby to play with. But all too often, we are trained as parents to freak out over a baby touching or holding something (like dirt). By making a big deal out of it, you will actually pique his curiosity to do it even more. Let him feel the textures, shapes or even dig his hands in the mud if he must. This is how he learns about his world. Just make sure he doesn't eat it or put something in his mouth that is unsafe.

15. Stimulating toys. Of course every baby loves toys. Choose toys that stimulate their minds. You can also play with your baby by making tunnels to crawl through out of blankets, playing peek-a-boo; getting a walker and other homemade ideas that will mentally stimulate your baby.

16. Make funny faces and act silly, using variable voice inflections, tones and noises. Mix it up. Talk to him sometimes as if he were an adult, but then other times in baby talk. Make funny faces and touch your baby. These things create a bond and will make your baby aware of the fact there are hundreds of ranges that can be expressed through one voice – yours.

17. Introduce your baby to more than one language. You may think it will confuse your baby, when in fact this is the best time to make your child bi-lingual.

18. Healthy eating. Although it may be tempting to give the baby chocolate, cookies and French fries, these offerings can lead to poor consequences, including slowing his mental development or inhibiting his physical attributes. Small pieces of fish, peas, blueberries and turkey are okay as your baby begins eating more solid foods. Your baby will learn to make healthy choices if that is what he is used to eating all along.

19. Keep your baby on breast milk or formula as long as possible. Doctors say you can begin weaning your baby as he nears the year mark, but milk has a ton of hormones and antibiotics that are injected by the dairy farmers. There are hundreds of studies now that prove the probiotics found in baby formula and in breast milk provide the much-needed nutrition for optimum development. Formula may be expensive, and milking is a hassle, but these are very valuable when it comes to your baby's early foundation for immunity.

20. If at all possible, try to get in-home care or a part time nanny instead of daycare. Kids these days pick up too many bad habits at daycare centers (not all, but a greater majority). Some are deprived of the one-on-one attention provided by adult stimulation because there are so many kids to take care of. Having a one-on-one provider for your baby means he will have all the attention to himself.

Subsequently, he will have more adult interaction and individual attention.

Yes, making your baby smarter takes work and is a never-ending task that you signed up for on the day the baby was born. However, now that life is no longer just about you and is instead about the life you created, now is the time to commit to and empower your baby while his mind is fresh; literally like a blank book with all of the pages just waiting to be filled to the brim.

Baby Exercise Tips

A recent BBC News article asked the question 'Are baby exercise classes the next big thing?' The article raised interesting points about the health and fitness concerns parents have for their babies in a climate of increasing childhood obesity and declining physical activity. Essentially, the article suggested that the earlier a baby was entered into a baby exercise routine, the less susceptible that child was to obesity and apathy. This guide offers some information and advice regarding baby exercise patterns.

Early-in-Life Exercise Routines

According to research by Sylvia Klein, an expert and prolific author on the subject of pregnancy and infant welfare, entering your baby into a movement programme or exercise regime increases the chances that your baby will talk earlier, eat better, sleep more restfully, and undergo faster development of their motor functions than a non-exercised baby. However, it's not necessary to pay out for expensive baby exercise classes, as the BBC's question implies. What follows is a short collection of ideas and tips to help you exercise healthily with your baby.

First, some general guidelines to remember:

Keep baby exercise sessions under half an hour each time, and don't exceed two sessions per day.

Speak to your doctor for ideas on which exercises to take part in. Not all baby exercise is appropriate for all infants, so talk with your GP about the ones which you would like to do.

Buy a mat or use a soft blanket to lay your baby on while you do the baby exercises.

Listen to your baby - if he or she is clearly unhappy with the exercises then stop.

Don't exercise a baby which has just eaten - that's asking for trouble.

Keep your movements relaxed and fluent. Don't force your baby's joints into position. You'll be surprised at how firm you can be, but don't make it uncomfortable.

Talk constantly and communicate with your baby - make the exercise fun and lively.

Exercise the joints which are closest to your baby's torso and radiate the movements outward; from the hip, to the knee, to the ankle, to the toes for example.

With these guidelines in mind, here are a few exercise ideas you can try at home. None of these cost anything to do, and they are designed to help you bond with your baby, while hopefully having some fun.

Pectoral & Chest Exercise

Lay your baby on his or her back and take each wrist or hand in yours. Stretch your baby's arms wide apart. Then bring your baby's hands all the way back across their chest so that their right hand is on their left shoulder and vice versa, and their little arms are crossed across their chest. Repeat this several times, applying pressure according to the strength with which your baby responds.

Hand to Opposite Foot

As the name suggest, this baby exercise involves contact being made between the left foot and right hand, or the right foot and left hand. With your baby lying on their back, bring their foot up to their opposite hand and hold them there for a few seconds. Then repeat with the other hand and foot. This is a good baby exercise for the back and the hips, and stretched big muscles in your baby's thighs and backside.

The Bicycle

Gently holding your baby by the lower legs or by the feet, rotate your baby's legs as though were cycling. Technically, a backwards-pedaling motion has the best effects. This is good exercise for the knees, hips, thighs and calves, and if you're holding your baby by the feet then their ankles will also be exercised. The back and bum will also benefit from this one.

The Sidekick

It's called 'the sidekick' because it describes the basic motions of this maneuver. Again with your baby lying on their back, bring their right leg out and across their left leg, as though they were kicking an imaginary football. Bring the leg far enough round so that the toes of the foot touch the mat or blanket they're lying on and the hip lifts slightly on its own. Repeat this several times and do the same for the other leg. This twisting motion is good for the flexibility and strength of many areas of the torso and legs.

Sit Ups

It is possible to train your baby to do full sit ups by laying them on their back, holding their feet down, and tempting them to sit up with food or toys. We don't advise this for everyone however, since most babies won't be strong enough. Instead, hold your baby by the hands and slowly lift them into a sitting position. If their neck is not yet strong enough to support the weight of their head, you will need to support it for them. Lower your baby back down to a prone position and repeat.

Baby Swimming & Yoga

Your baby will also benefit from exercise outside the house. Babies' instinct and comfort in the water is now pretty widely known, and most have heard of the 'dive reflex'. Swimming is great exercise for your baby's muscles and is generally a relaxing and fun atmosphere for the parents. We don't recommend swimming without expert guidance however, and there are classes at most gyms and leisure centres across the UK which will give you specialist advice and keep your baby safe.

CHAPTER SEVEN

Baby Sleep Help - Early Prep For Toddlerhood

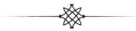

You're at your wits end, pulling out your hair, yawning all the time, and your eye lids feel the weight of the world. Instead of consistent sleep you are getting a couple of hours here and there because your baby cries for you throughout the night. You know you are not alone and you know this is all a part of parenting but what can you do to stop the interference of your sleep? How can you get your baby to sleep at night and through the night? Baby sleep help is a common need for new parents whose baby is out of the nightly feeding stage.

Put this baby sleep help into action tonight, but it is important to remember that consistency is what will solidify your child's nightly sleep pattern, and will be especially beneficial for you and your baby when they reach toddlerhood and preschooler years. Start early training for an independently sleeping toddler and preschooler by training your baby from now using the following tools.

A Solid, Warm, Cuddly Routine

As you may know by now babies feel more stable when they can get idea of what to expect next, which is why throughout the day it is preferred for many things to be handled on a routine basis. Getting your baby to sleep at night and throughout the night is no different.

Choose your baby's bedtime and begin the routine no later than 45 minutes before hand. Adjust the time if you need to but there should not be a lot of time in between each piece of the routine.It should flow together one after the other.

Calm, Cozy, quiet atmosphere. Turn the lights down and keep the noise down to a bare minimum.

Consider a baby massage as opposed to a bath. It offers health benefits, takes less time and effort, and is much more relaxing to you and your baby. Use this time to chat to your baby about the day and what exciting things they can expect tomorrow. Soft music and dim lights for a cozy atmosphere. No TV, no disruptions. All your attention should be focused on your baby.

Consider taking your baby directly to his room after his bath or baby massage, put him in his bed, and read him a story and sing a song (a relaxing tune).

It is here that common mistakes are made that can start bad habits causing sleep interruptions and major toddler and preschooler sleep problems.

If you rock your baby to sleep at night you are starting a pattern in which you nor your baby will be able to break, and you will find within a short time your baby cannot sleep without being rocked. He will wake up frequently, which is normal but he will need you to rock him back to sleep. This can go on and on unless you fix the problem. Do you have time as a parent and professional to undo things? Isn't it better to simply not let bad habits start? Of course.

Skip the rocking altogether and replace it with a bedtime story and songs in his comfy cozy room. This doesn't mean that you should never rock your baby. Rocking is enjoyed much by parent and child and of course is a wonderful time. You can rock with a story or songs during the day, morning, or early evening, well before bedtime. Just don't let it become a bedtime ritual that will later come to haunt you.

Bedroom Enhancements

Your baby's room should be ready in advance with a cozy, soft atmosphere.

A very soft night light so baby is not alone in the dark and can see the lovely things around him in his room.

My personal idea for a night light is a fish tank that your baby can see from his crib.

Soft music. If you can find something from his favorite baby show or cartoon it's preferred, but it should be soft, low key music.

Leave your baby's room door open when you leave the room and always tell him you love him and will check on him later. This is a phrase your baby should become familiar with by toddlerhood.

Give Baby Chances

Baby sleep help requires that you always give your baby a chance to fall asleep on his own. If he cries the minute you leave the room, give him a few minutes before you go rushing back in. Often times he will fall asleep on his own and this is good because it is preparing him for toddlerhood to be an independent sleeper which is what every parent wants! When you do enter his room adhere to the following:

Do not talk to your baby

Pat him on the back or stroke his head for a several seconds only (this is done to let your baby know that you are still around and have not completely left him).

Leave the room again and continue this process as needed, each time leaving a two minute gap in between the time you leave and re-enter the room. Add one minute more to each gap.

Nine out of ten times your baby will fall asleep before you need to go in for the second time. When he doesn't make sure he is okay with diaper wetness and that he is not ill. Otherwise, expect him to test your patience. It is then your responsibility to help him out and hold strong to the routine of the two minute gaps.

No matter how dreaded it seems to listen to your baby cry for a few minutes, rest assured it will not hurt him and what you are dreading now is nothing to what you will dread a short time later when they are in toddlerhood and can't sleep independently. If you begin doing this early, you will be doing yourself and baby a huge favor. Toddler and preschooler sleep help is much more dreaded because your baby is older and can walk and talk, adding more complications to parents when their toddler has a tantrum at bedtimes and won't sleep through the nights. Lack of sleep for you and your toddler massively disrupts many things including your child's learning abilities in school and their behavior throughout the day. A child with solid sleeping habits is a better behaved child with a better attention span and should be a part of your child's healthy lifestyle.

Daytime Prep

There are things you can do during the day toward baby sleep help. These things will help with your baby sleeping through the night.

Do not give foods that increase energy before bedtime.

Your baby should have a nap daily.

You should be supplying your baby a healthy diet, low in fatty foods.

Limit television watching to half an hour a day. You can increase this to one hour when baby gets a bit older.

Regular daily exercise appropriate for his age.

Put your baby on a sleep routine and stick to it on a nightly basis. Manipulate the routine to suit your child's age as he grows into toddlerhood. Help your baby to feel comfortable and secure in his room alone at night by providing him a nightlight and soft music, and do your best to avoid starting bad habits toward future bedtimes. With this baby sleep help you will be able to get your baby situated into a nightly routine to help you both now and in the future, and will help you avoid toddlerhood bedtime battles.

What Your Baby Needs From You in His First Two Years

Several new parents confuse in their first two years they have a new baby. Here's several things are important needs of children as they grow from birth into the first two years based on scientific studies and research.

1. Baby needs mothering being healthy and caressed, especially at feeding time.

2. New baby needs several hours of sucking a day.

3. He needs to be carried often to develop his sense of balance and his feeling of security.

4. Giving the baby prompt attention when he cries develops his sense of safety and trust

5. Singing, rocking, patting or holding your baby when his wakeful helps him sleep

6. A room of his own is important for baby's quiet and comfort and your own privacy

7. Needs frequent, open display of affection since he learns to love by being loved

8. Let him feed him self when he shows interest even though he makes a mess

9. Be sure your baby has room and opportunity for free movement and exploration

10. His first playthings should be ones that satisfy his need to handle, bang, suck, throw

11. Companionship and play with parents are important to any baby

12. Needs matter of fact parental attitude. Show no disgust at elimination.

13. With a little help a child toilet trains himself when he is ready.

14. Needs practice in talking and listening, to develop his ability to communicate.

15. Needs to have his parents realize that he is not a little adult.

16. A child needs to grow at his own pace and be appreciated-not pushed.

17. Needs a relaxed, responsive mother who plans rest and recreation for herself and her baby.

18. A cooperative, harmonious home atmosphere is important-tensions distress a baby

19. Needs to be given as much freedom as is sensible, not hedged in with Don'ts.

20. By asserting himself, he gains the sense of being an individual.

21. He also needs to fill that he is a member of a family group.

22. Among his needs are toys and materials he can master-not once he can't manage.

23. A child needs to be able and encouraged to display love for others.

24. He needs to consider all parts of his body as clean and acceptable.

25. The young child needs to climb, run, pull, be physically active.

26. He needs to play freely and be allowed to get dirty.

Baby Sleeping - Things To Remember About Your Baby's Sleep

Sleep is very important for your baby's early growth and development. However, you may find it hard to get your baby off to sleep or, she may slips naturally into good sleep habits. An infant cannot distinguish the difference between day and night. The usual sleep pattern of a typical baby during the first 2 months of life is to randomly sleep from 16 to 20 hours within a 24 hour cycle. If your baby is put to sleep awake frequently at the same time each night, the baby's sleep pattern will start to change and will be sleeping for longer periods when the baby reached 8 to 12 weeks old.

Baby Sleeping Difficulties

There are a lot of reasons that makes babies starts waking up during the night. It could have something to do with the temperature of his room, the lights and ventilation, or the noise present within your home or in the neighborhood. If so, try to fix the situation. Other reasons are illnesses or some developmental changes. For example, if your baby has learned a new developmental skill such as learning to crawl, he might want to try it out every chance he gets, even within his usual sleeping hours.

Baby Sleeping Guidelines

Every parent will have different stories to tell when talking about their newborn baby sleep patterns, some do in fact sleep like infants, while others seldom sleep through the night for a long time. Some babies are comfortable to soothe themselves until they sleep, while others want the lullabies of their parents, milk feeding or a comfortable crib to help them to sleep.

Self-Soothe Sleep

Most of baby sleep researches suggest that the most important step in teaching your baby to sleep through the night is to have him fall asleep on his own. According to research, this is the answer to prevent baby sleep pattern difficulties.

Feeding

In most cases, by the 10th to 16th week of your baby, if your baby has eaten enough food before going to sleep, he is more likely to awaken during the night expecting to be fed. According to research, it is suggested to help your baby learn to sleep through the night by giving him considerable feeding at the same time each evening, between 10 pm and midnight. In addition, feeding a baby after midnight can usually disturb his sleeping pattern.

Baby's Crib

Baby cribs are designed not only to complement your baby nursery's decor, but to also provide a safe, cosy place for your baby to sleep into.

With so many available styles and options on baby cribs today, purchasing the perfect baby crib can be a demoralising task. You have to make sure that the baby crib you are about to purchase meets the minimum quality standard. A safe baby crib must have a firm and fitted mattress, no missing or broken slats, and no sharp edges on all corners. Also, it is advised for parents to settle for the stationary side baby cribs rather than drop-gate cribs, because the later could present some serious baby safety issues.

How to Choose Baby Playpens That Are Comfortable For a Baby

If you are looking for a baby playpen, comfort should always count first. Just imagine your baby is delivered to this unfamiliar world which is surely a big contrary to his mother womb. He is so feared and at the same time curious about all the surroundings, all the noises and visions that come to his proximity.

How do we help this little angel to get with the human world? Besides being pacified by parent hugging, a nice sleeping playpen is an immediate solution to his fear. A comfortable playpen with warmth of family will surely helps a great deal.

Here, a nice playpen will mean a nice and comfortable womb to him, comparatively much look alike to a place that he feels a high sense of security and geniality. Choose a playpen that is sturdy to support the baby, and make the baby feel safe.

Especially for those playpens which meet all JPMA safety standards and requirements. Also choose a playpen that is set with comfortable cushions and quilting. Set the playpen with nice baby bedding, to make him feel extremely nice and warm in his little universe. Of course, organic fabric for baby bedding is most ideal, because it has the best texture and non-toxic materials. It could avoid causing any allergy to your baby when he is not yet strong enough to fight against the unnecessary bacteria and allergic elements.

Set the playpen with nice baby plush toys too to delight your baby. There are lots of plush toys with organic fabric. Find the playmates for your baby and to keep him accompanied by the tiny toys and dolls whenever it is his play time or sleep time.

Last but not least, there are lots of playpens are designed with special functions to provide extra comfort to baby. You will have portable musicals with funny toys to amuse the baby. By extending his little legs or hands to reach for the toys, these kinds of physical trainings will be good to the baby.

There are some mattresses mounted with vibrations, so that once the vibration is switched on, it will comfort your little one to have a beautiful sleep time, and there is no need for you to bribe him to sleep at all.

CONCLUSIONS

Infant sleep is a particularly interesting field of research due to its dynamic trajectories, the developmental changes that occur during this period, and the interaction with other developmental domains. More specifically, we reviewed the association between infant sleep and cognition as well as physical growth. From the reviewed literature, we conclude that sleep plays a key role in those domains with its maturation paralleling, preceding, as well as resulting from interactions with cognitive and physical maturation.

For future research, a combination of objective and subjective methods of sleep assessment is desirable, especially in the longitudinal exploration of both quantitative and qualitative aspects of sleep and infant development. From the cross-sectional studies, it is not possible to draw strong causal links between the two based on existing literature. For future studies, we propose to adopt a trajectory design which may reflect better the maturation and dynamic development, especially at young ages. It may furthermore improve the predictability of long-term effects on health and development compared to the predictability of cross-sectional time-point estimates as well as enabling us to examine the effects of cumulative sleep as compared to critical periods in the above relation. This is important to understand as sleep is one early life factor that can be targeted for interventions to optimize early development.